SECOND CHANCE

SURVIVING THE BATTLES OF CANCER!

Bayo & Yinka Oladele

WHAT PEOPLE ARE SAYING ABOUT "SECOND CHANCE"

"…This book will give inspiration and hope to other people battling with life threatening diseases.. We recommend this book for everyone…"

Pastors Ademola & Iheoma Farinu

"…As you read through the pages of this book, you will read of a man and his family…who trusted God completely with his life."

Rev. Noral Woodburn

"…It kept my attention as I read it. Telling your story will help…those battling cancer and the ones walking with them."

Mark Williams, Pastor

"…we can attest to the factuality of this book. This book is an empowering life story, and a must read for enlightenment…"

Daniel & Marian Ofiuvwo

"This book is a proof. The hope is that readers will be encouraged, strengthened and delivered from this deathly attack called Cancer. God is good!"

Dr. Adeyinka & Oluyinka Marcus

"This book is a must read. Reading about the concepts from a lived experience brings the meaning closer to home while helping to create hope."

Mr. Wale & Dr. (Mrs.) Juliet Onabadejo, RN

"The Auithor has provided insight to the fact that Faith and Science does not conflict…This is a must read book".

Mr. & Mrs. Temitope Esan

"The book shows the relevant place of both social and faith… We gladly recommend the book for your reading or gifting it to a friend in need of encouragement."

Dr. Abiodun & Caroline Coker

"This book will give you good understanding about cancer disease."

Pastors Tunde & Bose Aina

"The courage, candour and openness with which the Oladeles are dealing with the life-changing event is, in the very least, highly commendable and admirable "

Chief & Chief (Mrs.) Adeniyi & Lolade Akanni

"We often describe you as an open book and sharing your journey with cancer in this book attest to it." God bless.

Mr. & Mrs. Tumi & Kike Aderibigbe

"We will like to congratulate the family for the defeat of cancer in the life of our Brother, glory be to God!"

Pastors Fola and Sunny Adeniyi

"…this book, tries to assure readers that being diagnosed for cancer is no confirmation of "death warrant."

Mr. & Mrs.Phillip & Olubunmi Latilo

"This book is an educative, inspiring and poignant account of the reality of the cell compositions in the human body"

Mr. & Mrs. Derin & Moji Taiwo

"Reading this book gave us new eye sight similar to one who was blind and now could see."

Pastors Ben & Dee Adekugbe

"It is obvious that Bayo wrote this book in an effort to aid other cancer patients."

Mr. & Mrs. Peter & Julie Oganwu

"This will go a long way in motivating others to remain hopeful and be strong in the face of any traumatic experience."

Alhaji & Alhaja Azeez & Adenike Ola-Ojetola

"Permit me to call this book a story of courage and the testimony of how being tough can last tough time."

Pastors Samuel & Olufunke Ilesanmi

"Reading SECOND CHANCE lays out the biblical rationale for believing that God still actually heals today, and that He uses people of faith to bring His healing today."

Pastors Olatubosun & Monisola Sowunmi

"I encourage you all to read and enjoy and support the efforts of Bayo and Yinka, in this masterpiece – written from the hearts."

Dr. Julius Adekunle & Mrs. Elma Ogunnariwo

"We salute Mr. & Mrs. Oladele's courage to publish this book for the benefit of mankind."

Alhaji & Alhaja Muideen & Basirat Adeyemi

"This book is a great resource for the fight of faith, test of friendship and the bond of love."

Mr. & Mrs. Seun & Bukola Ogunsola

"God will never give you a test that is above you. I will encourage anyone who desires to be motivated in life should lay hands on this book."

Dr. Sam & Mrs. Tinu Anifowose

"I recommend this book to any one who wants to grow in faith, particularly those who are believing God for healing."

Rev. Kenny Thompson

"Interesting and educational. The information in the book must be shared with *(all)* that we can beat cancer."

Mr. & Mrs. Wale & Bernie Gbalajobi

"As you read this book ...we pray that your testimony will abide in Jesus Name."

Deacon Michael & Dr. (Mrs.) Lydia Oladosu

"...he fought and conquered the battle called cancer to the glory of God."

Mr. Sina & Mrs. Sola Akinsanya

"We are convinced that this book will surely encourage any one passing through same experience."

Dr. Theo & Mrs Uche Okeke

Library and Archives of Canada Cataloging in Publication:

Second Chance
Surviving the Battles of Cancer
ISBN: 978-1-7750542-0-7
Oladele, Bayo & Yinka
Calgary, AB Canada

Printed in Canada

DEDICATION

This book is dedicated to the glory of God, the creator of blood, bone, body and every part in our body, for giving me a second chance of life.

To Lekan & Zandra, families and friends - You showed me strength and reasons to live by your prayers, encouragements and support.

To Zoë, Grace, Ochaya, Ireayooluwa – You brought a new life into our family.

To all the survivors, fighters, deceased. caregivers and families of cancer patients everywhere.

To my dear wife and my co-author – I am alive today because of you, and because of the power of God that works life through you.

DEDICATION

CONTENTS

FOREWORD

An anthropologist interviewing the average person today will come to a startling conclusion: despite our societies' economic abundance, cultural opulence, and technological sophistication, many people think they are not getting enough satisfaction out of life.

When asked what is wrong, people point to different things: their bodies, personalities, jobs, bad habits, and so on. Nevertheless, improving how they feel about these parts of their lives doesn't necessarily make them feel more satisfied.

The essence of our lives is well captured in the definition of health by WHO, "A state of complete physical, mental and social well-being, and not merely the absence of disease or infirmity.

The authors of this book actually did justice to the above definition of health in narrating their experiences during diagnosis and treatment of Bayo's illness.

I have known this couple for over 15 years in our community; they are both examples of what we can refer to as good servants in our society. They do not only serve by giving their time, also, they give their resources and help others in the community. It is not surprising when the response to them during their trying period was very overwhelming. I had the unique opportunity of visiting them several times and being close to the couple during their hospital stay.

The idea of writing about their experiences during Bayo's hospital admission and the title chosen for the book, i.e. second chance, is well thought out. Going through the pages of the book, the way the content is arranged is impressive. The biopsychosocial nature of the illness is emphasized in the book, and the hints on how to navigate different challenges that accompany every stage of the illness is explained.

As mentioned above that the idea of writing this book is a bold one and commendable, many people will find it difficult to think of what has happened and the trauma that they went through during the treatment. The thought alone will be too much for them to bare, not to talk about writing. Being a psychiatrist myself, I have seen a lot of people that have developed posttraumatic stress disorder following diagnosis and the treatment received for an illness like this.

The authors attempted to demystify the diagnosis and treatment of cancer and also, emphasized the need to get an early diagnosis and be open to various forms of treatment offered for different conditions that they may have.

This book will be an easy read to understand how to go about seeking help for individuals or relatives of people diagnosed with cancer. Going through the treatment of cancer can only be well explained and narrated by people who have gone through it before.

The authors really understood that it was the grace of God that saw them through the ordeal of cancer, as a result, they decided to share their experience.

"And he said, I will make all my goodness pass before thee, and I will proclaim the name of the Lord before thee; and I will be gracious to whom

I will be gracious, and I will shew mercy on whom I will shew mercy." Exodus 33 vs 19.

Chief (Dr.) Samuel Oluwadairo, MD, F RCPC
Consultant Psychiatrist
Foothills Medical Centre, Calgary, Alberta

PREFACE

"Eni t'okan lo mo *(a Yoruba proverb)*"- "it is only those that are affected that know the impact" which in this case means "only the patient can tell...", or "He who feels the pain, understands the pain" is the summary of cancer treatment experience, and the same may be said for the primary caregiver. It's almost impossible to describe the real feeling of a cancer patient, especially during the critical periods of the treatments; and there are indeed many critical times for any cancer patient.

Most people who came to visit me, either at home or the hospital, knew one person or another, a family member, colleague or relative who is a survivor, a fighter or, deceased because of cancer. What many people do not know is where a patient can find genuine, and easy to read account of a survivor's experience. Something that is not too narrow to one particular form or area, and at the same time, contained reliable information.

In many cases, the emotion of the patient tends to colour and overshadow the message that the author was trying to convey or pass across. In other situations, the view will be skewed towards a sect, faith, or culture, which usually makes the focus of the book to be forgotten.

Cancer is no respecter of sex, faith, colour, culture, age or society. When we give an account of our ordeals and journey through victory, we need to include everybody as much as possible, while our individuality remains unshaken.

This book covers some preliminary information most people look for, either as a patient, a caregiver or as someone who is interested in cancer or cancer treatments. It gives a simple, clear and reliable information about cancer, its causes, and some signs and symptoms to watch out for. It might be important to state here that at the initial stages, signs, and symptoms that are characteristics of cancer can be mistaken for a non-cancer disease and vice versa. This is why it is advisable to seek an expert's opinion when you see a sign or experience a symptom.

Lastly, this book also offers an overview of the art of caregiving. It is important to note that caregiving is a thankless job, especially when the primary caregiver is a close relative of the patient. Caregivers require as much attention and support as the patient.

By having a clear mind, taking every sign and symptom seriously and acting on them at their early stages, and following the established and scientifically proven medical processes, we hope that certain cancers will soon be downgraded to a non-terminal chronic disease. It is my hope that this book will help to shed more light on the subject of cancer, and remove some of the superstitions around it.

The practical experience detailed towards the end of the book is to help readers "see" from the eyes of the patient, and to share in the patient's ordeal and by so doing, lifting some of the weights from his/her shoulder, for "a burden shared is a burden halved."

Our prayers are that none of us will ever pass through this kind of ordeal again. But if we have to, it will not be in utter darkness; we will have a manuscript for the road.

Bayo and Yinka Oladele
2017

ACKNOWLEDGMENT

We would like to acknowledge everyone who stood by us, prayed for us, visited the hospital and home, may God bless you richly – including but not limited to members of the Nigerian-Canadian Association of Calgary. The Yoruba Foundation of Calgary, Beddington Pentecostal Church (BP Church), RCCG House of David, Calgary, RCCG Christ Love Assembly, Christ Apostolic Church (Vineyard of Comfort), Worldwide Acceptance Ministries, Encounter International Ministry, Hope Alive Counselling, Calgary World Harvest, All Woman Ministry, Nigerian Muslims Congregation, Calgary (NMCC), staff members at The UPS Store #45, Princess of the Kings Prayer Group, Holy Ghost Encounter Prayer Group. Our families, siblings in-laws; children, friends, relatives, Dr. Peter Duggan, Dr. Nancy Zacarias and other doctors, pharmacists, nurses and staff of Foothills Medical Centre and Tom Baker Cancer Centre, and others too numerous to mention.

We acknowledge my big brother Mr. Debo Oladele. You dropped everything to be with me during my trial period.

We also acknowledge our reviewers and advisers for your relentless efforts toward the production of this book.

We appreciate and thank you very much for all your prayers, care and support during our trial period.

PART 1

THE NATURE OF CANCER

Second Chance – Surviving the battles of cancer

INTRODUCTION

No, in all these things we are more than conquerors through him who loved us. For I am sure that neither death nor life, nor angels nor rulers, nor things present nor things to come, nor powers, nor height nor depth, nor anything else in all creation, will be able to separate us from the love of God in Christ Jesus our Lord. Romans 8:37-39 (NIV)

Second Chance at Life: Surviving the Battles against Cancer

Cancer is still one of the most feared and dreaded of all diseases at present. This is very much a reality because according to the World Health Organization[1], there has been an alarming increase in the number of people currently suffering from different forms of

3

cancer; and the World Cancer Day[2] reported that millions of people have already been killed by this distressing disease.

Our body is made up of many billions of cells that make up the tissues, the organs, fluids and the bones. Generally, the cells undergo the process of continuous cell division, either to create new cells or to replace ageing cells, as cells typically die after a specified span of time.

However, when the cells divide in a pace that is different from the norm, and there is a mutation of the cells due to genetic changes, production of abnormal cells takes place. Some of these abnormal cells later come together to form a hard mass or tumour and cancer.

Being diagnosed with cancer has a great impact on the person's mental, emotional and psychological lives and eventually, the person needs to cope with it. Here are some ways to help a person cope with cancer:

1. Get as much detail about the condition
2. Be open to all treatment options
3. Learn to anticipate all major physical changes
4. Be prepared for lifestyle modifications and maintaining a healthy lifestyle

4

5. Ask for help and emotional support from family and friends

During treatment, you will need the help of a caregiver. The role of a caregiver will include the following:

1. To ensure that the patient is taking the necessary medications
2. To help through the adverse effects of treatments
3. To provide support, especially during the tough times

Being diagnosed with cancer is a bumpy journey, not only for the patient, but for the people who are involved in the care, the caregiver, family members, and friends. Battling cancer takes quite a long time because a patient goes through various stages of treatment, even into the remission period.

The entrance into remission is an indication that the patient has to a large extent, fought and overcame to a degree the cancer disease, at least for now. It also signals the beginning of a second chance at life. A rare opportunity to live again!

CHAPTER ONE

SECOND CHANCE

"Even though I walk through the valley of the shadow of death, I will fear no evil, for you are with me; your rod and your staff, they comfort me."Psalm 23:4

A second chance is a rare opportunity to do over, or redo something. Not so many people have the privilege and opportunity of a second chance, and not all those who have been given a second chance realize or understand it. And, when you do not recognize something, how can you appreciate it? Where there is no recognition, realization and/or appreciation, there can be no action!

The second chance is when you have literally lost everything, and you are powerless in the face of things around you, and your only option is to "reboot." When everything you have laboured for suddenly comes to a standstill, and there seems to be no way out but to start all over again!

Second Chance is when you make a career change deliberately or otherwise, as a result of changes in time and/or space.

Second Chance can be voluntary where changes in your life are as a result of your deliberate initiation, such as migrating from one place to another with the intent to start a new profession, career, or a new life. It can also be voluntary when, after a long life of work in a field or industry that has not particularly met your yearning or satisfied your desire in life, you decide to go back to school to study an entirely different course, applying to a different or new career.

Other things in life that bring second chances include weddings and marriages, the sudden demise of loved ones or breadwinners of families, natural disasters, certain illnesses, unexpected fortunes that bring increased lease of life and unimagined opportunities, and similar other things.

When the second chance is unexpected, or when it comes with little expectation, and particularly when the process by which it came about is positive and painless or with little pain, it's usually difficult to perceive it as such. Most times, we just accept it and move on with our lives, enjoying the unexpected fortune as an extension of our hitherto life, or as a reward for or the crowning of our previous or up-to-now efforts and struggles.

Weddings and marriages or re-marriage, especially after the loss of loved ones or at an old age, after a long wait, may be considered

> *"There is a message locking within you or your being that must be let out. Look deep within yourself, and the light of the soul – the Christ within – will reveal the hidden secret."*

as a second chance. The demise of a loved one or bread winner of a family usually leaves the family in a situation where all that has been done or left undone till the time of the demise is not only subject to review but to changes in some cases. Families are scattered, properties are sold, children dropped out of school, and everyone has to restart afresh. It is also a second chance, even when the situation seems dire and unfriendly; it is never-the-less an opportunity to start again!

Natural disasters have no respect for individuals, except for those who have taken into consideration, the potential for such event, and have built resistance into their lives. Only nature, in some seemingly bizarre, random and unexplained ways and some quick sense of response and alertness of some people, determine the survivors in major disasters. Even then, it's always a start over and a new beginning for almost everyone that survives.

Certain illnesses that are terminal have unusual ways by which they exact pain and suffering in the lives of the patients. Cancer, for example, can be an unexpected and a sudden affliction that summarily transforms the life of the patient within a couple of weeks such that, the patient is left completely confused in the least. With the possibility of a second chance, the patient builds up hope and sufficient energy to keep him/her 'afloat' and going.

How To Ascertain Second Chance beyond reasonable doubt.

Despite the persistent present situation, you should know and be convinced that you have been given a second chance when:

- In your dream or otherwise, you were "told" in no uncertain words that "the situation is not unto death, but that the glory of God might be manifested."
- You must go through all stages of the treatment for the experience and "future purposes," so as to be in the position of knowing and to understand.
- On occasions, you had to be literally stabilized or brought back to life:
  - By someone who only happened to be around at the auspicious moment.
  - Or by a group of nurses after serious rigor that left by-standing friends and relatives crying.
  - Or by a group of ICU doctors after several minutes of serious therapy and medication.
  - Or by other means and situations similar to these
- In spite of the bumps on the road, the rejections and delays, failures and setbacks, discouragements and disillusionments, you

11

are alive; you did not die, rather, you are succeeding and on the way towards achieving your goals.

To be accorded a second chance is not something to be taken with levity or carelessness. Not everyone has the privilege. The demands and responsibilities of a sacrosanct second chance are seemingly higher and greater than that of a normal life. If for no other reasons, you most likely don't have any other opportunity left and if you 'blow' this one, you are on your own!

With greater opportunities come greater responsibilities. Now, there is no room for excuses as before! It is up to you to find out what your responsibilities are, and to brace yourself up to meet them optimally.

If no other clue appears to you, you must realize the fact that you were able to go through the various stages of the treatments (or whatever your trying situation may be) and survived. There is a message locking within you or your being that must be let out. Look deep within yourself, and the light of the soul – the Christ within – will reveal the hidden secret.

CHAPTER TWO

CANCER

"Even though I walk through the valley of the shadow of death, I will fear no evil, for you are with me; your rod and your staff, they comfort me."Psalm 23:4 (NIV)

The Perception

The way cancer is usually discovered or diagnosed in most patients has created the perception, by many, that it is a mysterious disease. In the past, people diagnosed with cancer would die within a few weeks or months of diagnosis – cancer was then considered a death sentence irrespective of the type, time/age or place.

However, with the advent of science and technology, civilization and the marvelous achievements of the medical sciences, cancer diagnosis no longer means summarily death sentence. This good news must be spread to all corners of the world. People must be made to understand and believe that cancer is no longer an automatic and immediate death sentence.

Although the experiences of people who have survived the ugly "trial" of cancer may differ, people should openly declare their triumph in order to encourage and, in some cases, enlighten their community that THERE IS HOPE!

It is true, however, that people are still dying of cancer within few days, weeks or months of diagnosis even in most advanced and developed environments. This truth must be recognized, and indeed, this statement may never be totally overcome due to the complexities of human species such as superstition, fear, outright denial, ignorance, poverty, lack of right information and many others.

These complexities also range from things within our control to those things above and beyond the current science and civilization.

* * *

Cancer is like a woodpecker, but only more dangerous and much more deadly. A woodpecker bores holes in a tree to make homes or territories. Trees don't die from

> *"CANCER IS NO LONGER AN AUTOMATIC AND IMMEDIATE DEATH SENTENCE."*

woodpeckers' activity as they primarily act on dead wood and the living standing trees don't fall off because only a small portion of the tree is impacted or marked.

Unlike the woodpeckers of the wild, the "body's pecking birds of cancer" mistake the tissues and fluids of the body organs (livers, lungs, kidneys, hearts, intestines and colons, breasts, eyes, bones and marrows, brain, pancreas, testicles and ovary, the skin, throat, ear, and many others), for the trunks and stems, and shoots and branches of a tree. The objectives are not for shelter, but are usually for aggressive and hostile territorial usurpation. Cancer indiscriminately and eventually, when not checked, takes over the body of the host patient, and by so doing, killing the host and destroying itself. As demonstrated down the ages, the only objective of cancer is to destroy, to steal and to kill.

* * *

Why cancer diagnoses look like A death sentence

In most cases, cancer is not diagnosed until it has crossed the stage of no return. These are dramatic situations where the diagnosis of cancer in a seemingly healthy person before the diagnosis, turns awry the moment after diagnosis. This is because, before the diagnoses, the spreading of the cancer cells has either not crossed a particular threshold, or important organs have not yet been affected. Since cancer, from my deductions, is *really not a disease*, but an inordinate and uncontrolled multiplication and spreading of previously good but now malformed and malignant cells.

As an illustration, a living tree that is being cut will not wither or fall until a substantial portion or vital parts of it have been hewed. It may continue to live and even flourish as long as certain thresholds that sustain the tree are intact. Anyone looking at the tree from a far distance would never know the tree was about to fall.

In a like manner, a seemingly perfectly healthy person that is carrying cancer cells around may not know or show any major signs or symptoms as long as the cells have either not attacked a major organ, a small part of an organ is affected but not enough to cause damage, or a certain threshold has not been crossed.

Just as crossing certain thresholds on a tree being cut may lead to withering, so could the discovery of cancer lead to serious illness, and near-death experiences. Furthermore, just as crossing other thresholds when cutting a tree

> *"Just as crossing other thresholds when cutting a tree may lead the tree to fall immediately and without notice, so could the discovery of cancer lead to a sudden and unexpected death of the patient."*

may lead the tree to fall immediately and without warning, so could the discovery of cancer lead to a sudden and unexpected death of the patient.

As a survivor, my understanding of cancer is that every person is a potential cancer patient because:

- We all carry potential cancer cells in our bodies.

- Every organ, every fluid, every tissue, every bone, every part and every cellular structure in our body has a potential to grow into cancer.
- Cancer is no respecter of anybody.

What is cancer?

It was about 5:30 pm Mountain Time on March 28, 2016, my wife and I were waiting eagerly for the result of the doctors' finding. I sat at the edge of the bed, while my wife was busy with her smartphone. I later discovered that she was trying to decipher the small information the doctor could divulge!

"It looks like myeloma..." said the doctor, "...but we need to wait for the oncologist's assessment," the doctor had concluded. Oncologist! That is a Cancer doctor! But Myeloma, what do they mean and what does it mean to me, I wondered silently?

While I was pondering over the doctor's statements, my wife was already on the internet searching for the meaning of the new terminologies that will continue to be an integral part of the rest of my life! My file was passed on to the Cancer clinic, the Tom Baker Cancer Centre, and I was asked to come back in two days, Wednesday, March 30, to meet with the Oncologist.

Within these two days and for many more days and months that followed, I did an extensive research on cancer and its symptoms, and why it seemed to have come on me so suddenly.

* * *

"Cancer is a group of diseases involving abnormal cell growth with the potential to invade or spread to other parts of the body."[3, 4]

Simply put, cancer is like a canker that eats into the body system of the host, the infected or the patient. It thrives on, steals, kills and destroys everything in its path. Cancer is merciless, respects nobody, and it's discovery in a person

> "Cancer is an unusual occurrence of the otherwise normal situation in the human body."

is often like a pronouncement of a death sentence.

But we are already aware of this morbid fact. What is it then that we do not know about cancer? Why is it so mystifying, and why do many people still today, feel frightened or scared of even mentioning its name?

In the recent days, I've met people who would rather refer to cancer as "that thing," "the C," etc.!

Cancer isn't a single disease, according to 'The American Association for Cancer Research' (AACR). The term cancer encompasses more than 200 diseases, which are all characterized by the uncontrolled proliferation of cells. Ignoring the body's signal to stop malignant cells multiply and form tumours in organs and tissues.

It as an abnormal biological growth, which is a deviation from the intended, the norm and the expected, and from the normal processes.

Cancer is, therefore, an unusual occurrence of the otherwise normal situation in the human body.

"In a healthy body, cells grow and divide in a controlled, orderly fashion to replace those that have grown old or have been damaged and die by design in a process called apoptosis. Cancer occurs when these natural processes go awry." (AACR) [5, 6]

From the Canadian Cancer Society[7], we read that cancer is a disease that starts in our body cells. Our bodies are made up of billions and billions of cells, grouped together to form tissues and organs such as, muscles and bones, the lungs and the liver. The genes inside each cell order it to grow, work, reproduce and die. By default, our cells obey these instructions and we remain healthy. But sometimes, the instructions get mixed up, causing the cells to form lumps or tumours, or spread through the bloodstream and to other parts of the body.

Cancer is therefore, integrally a part of us. We all carry it around in one form or another[8, 9]. When managed rightly with the controlled duplication of cells, we are without cancer and cancer-free. When the cells are not controlled, abnormal growths occur and cancer results!

* * *

Multiple Myeloma

I was officially diagnosed with Multiple Myeloma on March 30, 2016.

Multiple Myeloma (MM) is a type of the blood cancers called cancer of the plasma cells.[10] Plasma cells are particular type of white blood cells that are found in the bone marrow and are responsible for producing antibodies.

MM is also called the cancer of the bone and bone marrow because the infected plasma cells formed tumors in the bone marrow leading to bone lesion.

There is no identifiable cause for multiple myeloma other than deformity in plasma cells.[11,12] The following table from Wikipedia summarized the characteristics of multiple myeloma.

The characteristics of multiple myeloma

Synonym	Plasma cell myeloma, myelomatosis, Kahler's disease
Specialty	Hematology and oncology
Symptoms	Bone pain, bleeding, frequent infections, anemia
Complications	Amyloidosis, kidney problems, overly thick blood
Duration	Long term
Causes	Unknown
Risk factors	Alcohol, obesity
Diagnostic method	Blood or urine tests, bone marrow biopsy, medical imaging
Treatment	Steroids, chemotherapy, thalidomide, stem cell transplant, bisphosphonates, radiation therapy
Prognosis	Five-year survival rate 49% (USA)
Frequency	488,200 (affected during 2015)
Deaths	101,100 (2015)

Wikipedia.org/wiki/Multiple_myeloma

Causes of cancer

From the various extracts and definitions discussed earlier, we can safely conclude that the causes of cancer are really NOT unknown! Cancer is **caused** by the uncontrolled abnormal growth of cells. What is not known, one may say, are the reasons behind these causes, or in other words, what is responsible for the uncontrolled abnormal growth?

"It is not generally possible to prove what caused a particular cancer because the various causes do not have specific fingerprints."[13]

In Table 1: Causes of Cancer below, we have the known causes and the true unknown causes:

1. Cancer is caused "by the uncontrolled proliferation of cells."[14, 15, 16] Why can we not control or prevent this proliferation?
2. When "the instructions get mixed up, causing the cells to form lumps or tumours." What is causing the natural biological instructions by the human body to the cells to get mixed up?

25

What is known	The unknown	Question / Comments.
Cancer is caused "by the uncontrolled proliferation of cells."	What is causing the proliferation of the cells?	Why have we not been able to control or prevent this proliferation?
It results when the instructions to the cells get mixed up.	What causes the instructions to the cells to be mixed up or messed up?	How can we prevent the unintended mix-up or corruption of the instructions to the cells?
An abnormal growth of cells.	What causes the cells to grow abnormally?	Do all abnormally growing cells lead to cancer? If not, why do some become cancerous while some do not?

Table 1: Causes of Cancer © Bayo Oladele

In a standard environment, we know that "what you sow is what you reap" or the input determines the output. When a system gets a wrong command, or a wrong instruction, the output, if any, will be different from the usual. In the same token, when the instruction is correct and right, the output is expected to be in conformance with the norm. What can, therefore, make the instructions to change by itself?

3. "Cancer is a group of diseases involving abnormal cell growth." Therefore, all cancers are caused by abnormalities or mutations in the DNA of cells in the body. What causes the abnormality in the growth of the cells? What causes the cells of the body to grow in an uncontrolled way?

Let's take a step back to examine a few more of the conditions around these causes leading to cancers.

The World Health Organization's cancer agency: the International Agency for Research on Cancer (IARC)[17] and the USA National Toxicology Program (NTP)[18], have different ways by which they classify potential cancer-causing situations.

For example, IARC, in its monograph, uses four classes to describe the potential causes of cancer in humans.

See Table 2: Cancer Causing Situations below.

It might be deduced from this table that the main cause of cancer is an exposure to certain potential cancer-causing substances.

Classification	Potential Cancer causing situation
1	Exposure causes cancer
2	Exposure probably or possibly causes cancer
3	Scientists are unable to determine or classify whether exposure does or does not cause cancer
4	Exposure probably does not cause cancer

Table 2: Cancer Causing Situations - Adapted from IARC Monograph

But is that all?

Classifications 3 & 4 worth further examination:

- In a situation where science cannot determine whether or not exposure was the cause of cancer, where else can we look for answer?

- And where we emphatically know that cancer was not caused by exposure, what is the next step? These lead me to the following potential alternative cause.

* * *

An Alternative (Probable) Cause of Cancer

A potential, non-conventional and "out of the box" look at cancer.

"Growth is the process of developing or maturing physically, mentally, or spiritually."[19] Every stage of growth has its set of conditions and rules - written and unwritten; its modes of operation and means of interaction.

When a person moves from one stage of natural development to another, he naturally drops some set of attributes, and picks up a whole new set that defines and governs the new stage.

If a person decides to bring the entire attribute and character of a younger, lower or previous stage of life to his new, higher or older stage, he will discover that he cannot operate and will be perceived as someone who is not ready, not mature or is incapable of the new life. At the same time, there are certain qualities and aspects of life that need to, and must be carried along as we progress in life.

In other words, when you move from one life stage to another, or when you are promoted or graduate from one school of life to another,

> *"Could cancer be caused by not letting go of an old habit, behaviour or thought?"*

you'll take with you all the lessons learned, and qualities acquired that will become the foundation for the new phase of life you just started. The glories and fruits of the previous phase become the bedrock of the new phase.

Many times, we try to carry everything that we had and used in our previous phase of life into our new life! We forget that each and every new life or phase has it's own specific rules, requirements, and expectations. Certain things are required to accompany you to your new phase, but a whole lot are expected to be left behind. That is one of the purposes of advancement and promotion - to shed old and worn out robes, materials and properties, and to acquire and don new ones, to drop and rid ourselves of old habits, characters and way of life, and imbibe new ones.

What would you imagine will happen when we fail to drop an old habit, or fail to learn the required new rules in a new environment?

Could cancer be caused by not letting go of an old habit, behaviour or thought?

Could cancer be caused by not being able to adapt to new conditions, new challenges, new requirements, new callings, etc. or a new environment; whether that environment is real or virtual, or the requirements are written or unwritten?

In other words, could cancer be caused by what we leave undone, or do in excess, or too well? Bottled up emotions, feelings, anxieties, fear, hatred, anger, jealousies, envy, lust, misplaced love, nepotism, egotism, and the emotions get transformed into or manifested in one form of growth (or tumour) or another. This is just like the energy that cannot be destroyed, but only transformed from one form to another.

31

If it were possible to link our habits, characters, emotions, feelings, fears, anger, laughter, happiness, ecstasy and other such emotional states and activities of a person to the cell behaviours, it might be possible to determine the nature and conditions of our body cells when we are manifesting any of these feelings.

For example, could long and protracted inhibition of a particular type of energy lead to or express itself in the unintended proliferation

> *"...could long and protracted inhibition of a particular type of energy lead to or express itself in the unintended proliferation of another energy or cell?"*

of another energy or cell? Could too much of a particular energy or unintended energy acting on certain body cells cause them to multiply indiscriminately, proliferate or metastasis?

"Energies follow thought" is a popular axiom. Could it be that the energies following or generated by some of our thoughts, especially those ones that we think are not effective, that we don't pay enough attention to or that we discount as jokes, fables or impossible, eventually manifest in the form of these unintended situations?

Regardless of whether these assumptions are true or not, it is always better to err on the side of caution and of good. Therefore, let us think more positively, and more inclusively, and maybe one day, our positive and inclusive thoughts will cancel out the potentially prevailing negative energies.

*　*　*

Types of Cancer

As indicated earlier, "Cancer is a group of diseases that involve abnormal increases in the number of cells, with the potential to invade or spread to other parts of the body." There are over 100 different types of known cancers and much more, depending on your sources, that affects the human body." [20, 21, 22]

It might be easier to categorize cancer in terms of it's nature, and according to the affected body part. There are groups of cancers that affect the body structures and the frame or the skeleton, which is evidenced by flesh and tissue cancers, intestine cancers, body organ cancers, body fluids cancers, and those that cross these categories and affect the combinations of body, forms, organs, structure, etc.

A comprehensive list of the types of cancer can be obtained from the various online sources, institutes for cancer research, and from the cancer centres all over the world.

At the Tom Baker Cancer Centre (TBCC), Calgary, Alberta, a snapshot of the most common types of cancer is on display. Free resources are also available at the TBCC Library for almost all the different types of cancer.[23]

Cancers are usually named after/from the organs or tissues of origin and formation. For example, lung cancer starts in the cells of the lung, and brain cancer starts in the cells of the brain.[24]

Cancers may also be described by the originating cells, that is the type of cell that formed them.

It is impossible to include the complete list of the types of cancer in a booklet like this one. An abridged list from the American Cancer Society is included below.

Types of Cancer:

Acute Lymphocytic Leukemia (ALL) in Adults	Lung Carcinoid Tumor
Acute Myeloid Leukemia (AML)	Lymphoma
Adrenal Cancer	Lymphoma of the Skin
Anal Cancer	Malignant Mesothelioma
Basal and Squamous Cell Skin Cancer	Melanoma Skin Cancer
Bile Duct Cancer	Merkel Cell Skin Cancer
Bladder Cancer	Multiple Myeloma
Bone Cancer	Myelodysplastic Syndromes
Brain and Spinal Cord Tumors in Adults	Nasal Cavity and Paranasal Sinuses Cancer
Brain and Spinal Cord Tumors in Children	Nasopharyngeal Cancer
Breast Cancer	Neuroblastoma
Breast Cancer in Men	Non-Hodgkin Lymphoma
Cancer in Adolescents	Non-Hodgkin Lymphoma in Children
Cancer in Children	Non-Small Cell Lung Cancer
Cancer in Young Adults	Oral Cavity and Oropharyngeal Cancer
Cancer of Unknown Primary	Osteosarcoma
Castleman Disease	Ovarian Cancer
Cervical Cancer	Pancreatic Cancer
Chronic Lymphocytic Leukemia (CLL)	Penile Cancer
Chronic Myeloid Leukemia (CML)	Pituitary Tumors
Chronic Myelomonocytic Leukemia (CMML)	Prostate Cancer

Colorectal Cancer	Retinoblastoma
Endometrial Cancer	Rhabdomyosarcoma
Esophagus Cancer	Salivary Gland Cancer
Ewing Family of Tumors	Skin Cancer
Eye Cancer	Small Cell Lung Cancer
Gallbladder Cancer	Small Intestine Cancer
Gastrointestinal Carcinoid Tumors	Soft Tissue Sarcoma
Gastrointestinal Stromal Tumor (GIST)	Stomach Cancer
Gestational Trophoblastic Disease	Testicular Cancer
Hodgkin Lymphoma	Thymus Cancer
Kaposi Sarcoma	Thyroid Cancer
Kidney Cancer	Uterine Sarcoma
Laryngeal and Hypopharyngeal Cancer	Vaginal Cancer
Leukemia	Vulvar Cancer
Leukemia in Children	Waldenstrom Macroglobulinemia
Liver Cancer	Wilms Tumor
Lung Cancer	

<u>www.cancer.org/cancer/all-cancer-types</u>[25]

* * *

Signs and symptoms of cancer

Why does cancer seem so elusive to discovery, until it is almost too late, for some people? Also, certain cancers show no apparent signs or symptoms, yet, once diagnosed, it seems to degenerate fast? Why does a seemingly healthy person, becomes a mortally sick individual immediately after diagnosis? Have the signs and symptoms been overlooked or not

> *"Signs and symptoms are external manifestations of internal activities that may or may not be recognized by anyone."*

appreciated for what they are? Is it true that "Cancer cells are found only when they are ready/make themselves available to be discovered, or when they want to be found?"

One of the best resources for concise information on signs and symptoms of cancer is the American Cancer Society, (ACS)[26]. The ACS contains a compendium of information on cancers, the types of cancer, the supposed causes of cancers, and the signs and symptoms of different types of cancer.

Signs are signals that can be seen or recognized by another person, while symptoms are signals that are felt or noticed by the individual who has it, but may not be readily visible to anyone else.

For the purpose of our discussion, the following definitions from the Merriam-Webster dictionary throw more light on the meaning of signs and symptoms[27]:

1. *Anything material or external that stands for, or signifies something spiritual:*
2. *Anything indicating the presence or existence of something else:*
3. *An objective evidence of plant or animal disease.*

Therefore signs and symptoms are external manifestations of internal activities that may or may not be recognized by anyone. They help us to know that something may be going on beneath the surface.

* * *

Common signs and symptoms of cancer

Like other diseases, cancer has several signs and symptoms[28] that may help people to suggest the possibility of cancer. The challenge is that signs and symptoms indicating a potential cancer are in some cases, the same as signs and symptoms of other non-life threatening or non-terminal diseases.

For example, we all have different pain at different times and in various parts of our bodies, and all of us have experienced one form

"Signs and symptoms are your friends! Look at yourself and if you see a sign, act on it!"

of pain treatment or another. Some of us have even gone through different types of therapy to diagnose the cause(s) of the pain, and to obtain a lasting solution. As we speak, some of us have pain in one part of our body or another, and many of us are on pain pills or medication. The question is, how do you know when an ordinary neck or ankle pain, for example, is no longer just pain, even when x-ray fails to show anything out of ordinary? You simply don't!

Signs and symptoms are your friends! Look at yourself and if you see a sign, act on it! Don't cover it up, don't ignore it, don't discount or discard it, and don't delay. If you see a sign or notice a symptom, act on it. Act on it by telling your doctor. You never know when a regular blood work may reveal a serious hidden symptom.

There are arguably very many different types of signs and symptoms of cancers. Some can be obvious and easy to discern, while others are vague and not so conspicuous.

From my experience and discussions with other cancer survivors, and statements or comments by professionals - when you see a sign or a symptom, please act on it immediately. Do not procrastinate, especially about what you don't know much about.

There are signs and symptoms that are common or shared by many cancers, and there are other signs and symptoms that are unique to each cancer. Some of these common signs and symptoms are listed below. A more comprehensive list of signs and symptoms is impossible to be listed in a booklet like this one.

Please note that, though these list are sourced from different reputable databases, they do not in any way constitute or replace a medical advice from a certified oncologist/doctor. Please consult your doctor when you see a sign or notice a symptom.

* * *

List of Cancer Symptoms

Cancer symptoms may be similar to or different from other chronic diseases or common symptoms. In my case, I had pain in my leg and lower back. However, the thought of back or leg pain leading to cancer was the last thing on my mind!

According to the National Cancer Institute[29], Cancer can cause many different symptoms.

Some of these include:

- Skin changes, such as:
  - o A new mole or a change in an existing mole
  - o A sore that does not heal
- Breast changes, such as:

- o Change in size or shape of the breast or nipple
- o Change in texture of breast skin
- A thickening or lump on or under the skin
- Hoarseness or a cough that does not go away
- Changes in bowel habits
- Difficult or painful urination
- Problems with eating, such as:
- o Discomfort after eating
- o A hard time swallowing
- o Changes in appetite
- Weight gain or loss with no known reason
- o Abdominal pain
- o Unexplained night sweats
- Unusual bleeding or discharge, including:
- o Blood in the urine
- o Vaginal bleeding
- o Blood in the stool
- Feeling weak or fatigued

The majority of the symptoms listed above are regular or daily occurrence, and do not necessarily mean that the patient has cancer - please always consult with your doctor.

CHAPTER THREE

COPING WITH CANCER

Therefore we do not lose heart. Though outwardly we are wasting away, yet inwardly we are being renewed day by day. For our light and momentary troubles are achieving for us an eternal glory that far outweighs them all. 2 Corinthians 4:16-18 (NIV)

The life of a cancer patient cannot be imagined by anyone else. The daily living and the well-being of a cancer patient can only be known by a fellow patient or caregiver. Coping with cancer is a very strenuous effort, one that affects all aspects of the patient's life and the lives of those around him/her including caregivers, family members, and friends.

Cancer is different from other diseases as the science only knows the beginning! Even with a good prognosis, what is known is the beginning and the point in time, because no one knows exactly what may follow! Unlike most other diseases and sicknesses, it's very difficult if not impossible for an oncologist to categorically declare the complete eradication of the cancer cells. So, even when a cancer cell is declared completely removed from a patient's body, the patient remains under the weight of the potential

> *"It's very difficult if not impossible for an oncologist to categorically declare the complete eradication of the cancer cells."*

presence or reoccurrence of the cancer cells. This is a reason why the term remission is used, rather than cure! In this type of situation, how does a person/patient live? How do the caregivers, family members, friends, and well-wishers relate with the patient and with themselves?

My experience and discussions with other cancer survivors showed that cancer, in addition to the apparent effect on the patient, can break a family, turn a family into a pauper and lead to stress among other side effects.

How then does a cancer patient cope with life, and how will the family and the caregivers cope with the situation? Some of the more obvious areas of challenges are considered in the following pages.

Common side effects of cancer

Some of the common side effects of cancer treatments include:

- Anemia
- Loss of appetite
- Bleeding and bruising
- Constipation
- Delirium
- Diarrhea
- Fatigue
- Hair loss
- Infections
- Memory or concentration problems
- Nausea and vomiting
- Nerve problems (Peripheral Neuropathy)
- Pain
- Sexual and fertility problems
- Skin and nail changes
- Sleep problems

Coping Financially

Money is undoubtedly one of the things that must be present, and be readily available for a successful cancer treatment. Demand for money shows up in different forms and times, and each demand must be adequately met and satisfied. Irrespective of your location, money is mandatorily required. Depending on your location, the amount of money needed at any time may vary. The baseline requirement is to have one form of insurance coverage or

"No one saves for the advent of a terminal disease."

another. A national, provincial, or state sponsored health (care) insurance is very important as much as possible.

Where one form or another of government health insurance is available, it rarely covers all aspects of cancer treatment. In most cases, a supplemental insurance coverage becomes essential. The supplemental health insurance can be from your place of work, or privately arranged with reputable insurance companies. Cancer treatment is very expensive, and any form of a genuine insurance coverage will be beneficial in alleviating potential financial crisis and stress.

There are situations where none or very few of these options are available to a patient. In such a case, potential third party funding or sponsorships should be investigated or pursued. Again, depending on your environment and location, eligibility criteria and other functions, the list of potential donors and sponsors will vary. In the majority of cases, donors usually sponsor small household items such as, transportation to and from the hospital, caregiver or support services, etc. However, bigger items like the cost of treatments and drugs are usually covered by the government or insurance companies.

In some cases, the cost of drugs and other big ticket items may be sponsored in part by donors.

Individual savings is also very critical, and goes a long way towards cancer treatment. In fact, in several cases, personal savings is usually the first call before insurance starts to kick in if the patient is fortunate or wise to have planned for any medical emergencies.

Since no one saves for the advent of a terminal disease, personal savings are usually not enough; and if it does, you will be left with little or nothing at the end of the treatment. Please discuss your financial situation with your oncologist, local cancer centre medical team, social workers, cancer online support groups, and other local similar groups. You never know where the help may come from!

I am privileged to be living in a country that not only provides medical support for it's citizens, but also cares tremendously about the well-being of the people. Canada's health system may not be the best in the world, but it is certainly not among the least. When it comes to cancer, Canada is one of the 11 countries that have a mortality rate[*] below 10 percent. See World Health Organization's World Health Statistics 2017: Monitoring health for the SDGs *(Sustainable Development Goals)*[30]. Most of the big ticket or high-cost cancer drugs were covered by the provincial health system, the Alberta's Health Services (AHS)[31], and the Tom Baker Cancer Centre (TBCC)[32].

I am also privileged to be working for a company, Canadian Pacific Railway[33], that has a long history of providing medical support for it's employees. The cost of other drugs that are

___

[*] Probability of dying from any of CVD, cancer, diabetes, CRD between age 30 and exact age 70 k (%)

48

not directly cancer drugs, (for example, drugs used to treat side effects of cancer drugs e.g. neuropathic pain) was partly covered by my company's health insurance.

These coverages, plus some generous donations from friends significantly alleviated the demand on our savings.

Some of the expenses to be aware of are:

- None cancer drugs not covered by any of the insurance coverages you may have.
- The cost to change your wardrobe as your physical appearances (weight, hair, etc.) change.
- The cost of potential changes in diet.
- Transportation, to and from, the several medical appointments.
- The potential cost of a caregiver.
- The cost of maintaining your home and your family will not diminish because of your situation.
- The usual bills including mortgages or rent, utilities, car payment, insurance, and other bills.

Coping Materially

Material needs and requirements during cancer treatments vary and differ for each cancer patient. Coping materially may be dependent on:

- Financial resources – as discussed in the previous section.
- Patient's freedom or mobility.
- The usual day to day need or Activities of Daily Living (ADLs)[34, 35]

Material needs, like most other things, do not stop just because one is undergoing cancer treatment. The mundane needs of a patient remain unchanged, and in many cases, increased because of alterations in conditions, circumstances and other things.

There might be need for a change in wardrobe, as a result of changes in the body physiology as mentioned earlier. This type of change would not only require financing, but also a caregiver, the person to arrange for them. In my case, I had to change some of my clothes; especially after the transplant. I lost a lot of weight and most of my clothes became too big.

Keeping your home in a state, that does not advertise sickness or show that someone in the house/home is incapacitated, is another measure that can help.

You must also ensure your children are catered for and attended to as required, and your other dependents are not left *in the cold* without proper attention.

Depending on your situation, physical exercise forms an essential part of both the treatment and recovery. You need to know what type of exercise is suitable for you, and obtain a workable professional schedule. This includes timing, exercise partner, or caregiver, or support person. It is reviving to get out of the house and go to the neighborhood playground, nearby park, or malls for a walk.

* * *

Coping Spiritually

One thing that needs to be realized is that cancer is both a physical and spiritual disease and as such, must be met and fought on both the physical and spiritual planes. The doctors have been able to successfully meet the medical aspect of the physical need based on the approved procedures and drugs.

Though, it may not be visible to the naked eyes, medical and scientific methods are still regarded as physical as they deal only with the physically seen or proven aspects, though through non-gross-physical method! An example is a cell that has been seen and confirmed to split autonomously without any catalyst or known physical agent.

The spiritual aspect is more complex for various reasons, some of which are obvious. Faith in the Creator, or in someone greater and more powerful than the patient, tremendously helps while coping with the cancer treatment or any other chronic disease. This is good because "faith is the substance of things hoped for *and* the evidence of things not seen." Heb. 11:1 (kjv)

Cancer treatment can be lonely. Finding solace in the creator and pouring out your mind even when everything else looks bleak, can strengthen you emotionally and spiritually.

Depending on your faith or religious background, below are some spiritual practices that may help you cope with your cancer, and it's treatments:

- Praying alone or with someone else
- Having someone else pray for you
- Meditation
- Meditative breathing
- Reading the Scripture or other holy books
- Saying one passage from the holy book over and over again
- Praying in tongues
- Praying in the language of your religion.
- Listening to classical or spiritual music
- Talking about spiritual matters with another person
- Reciting spiritual or holy mantras
- Singing praise songs and hymns

* * *

Spiritual (Faith) Challenges

Because our environment and the system do not expressly recognize or support faith-based and other spiritual therapy, psychosomatic[†] and allied therapies have been used in their place to fill the treatment gap. While significant advancements have been made in the treatments of psychosis, neurosis and somatic-related issues, the public recognition of the faith and other faith-based therapies may further enhance the current gains in the psychosomatic areas.

> *"The object of your faith will determine the strength and duration of your perseverance."*

Questions would remain, however, about when and where to stop, and how to identify the legitimate faith claims since the fundamental definition of faith preclude hard, scientific and physical evidence: "faith is the substance of things hoped for and the evidence of things not

---

[†] of, relating to, involving, or concerned with bodily symptoms caused by mental or emotional disturbance - https://www.merriam-webster.com/dictionary/psychosomatic

seen." Heb. 11:1. Faith is based on trust and the potential result which may or may not be due to the exercise of faith itself! It is, therefore, difficult to prove the efficacy of faith in the crucible of science!!

It seems that the acceptance of faith and religion in the public domain is limited to social-political correctness and to take care of certain rites.

Faith is one of the principles of life that cuts across all religions and schools of thought to a small or large extent. Everyone believes in something. The object of your faith will determine the strength and duration of your perseverance. It is a strong act of faith to say to oneself and repeatedly that "I shall not die, but live..." Psalm 118:17 in the midst of pains that are beyond description or when everything else looks impossible.

One question that keeps coming to mind in dire situations like this one is: why did God allow it to happen?

One simple answer is that it is a test of faith! Now and then, we fall into challenging situations just to build us up and strengthen our faith in God.

Another way of looking at it may be that it is not God, but ourselves that allowed it. God is infallible, and he is no respecter of persons. His laws are immutable and resolute from the beginning of times. When we contravene the laws, there are consequences. That does not necessarily mean we are sick just because of our sins.

Just as electricity is no respecter of anyone. It is an obedient and faithful servant when properly used. It can be a merciless master when handled inappropriately or with ignorance. But it can also be deliberately used to destroy.

Irrespective of the cause or reason behind a sickness, there is always Grace and Mercy of Christ for those who know. "My grace is sufficient for you" 2 Cor. 12:9 (kjv)

*   *   *

Potential (Mental/Spiritual) Side Effects of Cancer Drugs

Some of the cancer treatment drugs come with serious side effects that may include sleeplessness, nervousness, and mental confusion leading to erring thoughts and a confused state of mind.

When pain is one of the cancer symptoms, patients are usually prescribed strong painkiller drugs, most of which are narcotic drugs with extreme side effects that may include delusion, mental confusion, and nervousness.

When you cannot sleep at night or when you suddenly become frightened by previously familiar and ordinarily harmless places and situations; When untoward thoughts come your way, when the mind faces delusions, or when everything around becomes confused, , you should know that these are some of the effects and the pranks of the many narcotic drugs you've been using working on your mind. You need to talk to your doctor immediately.

Depending on your situation, you may be asked to stop the offending drug. The doctor may also prescribe another narcotic drug as a remedy!

Towards the end of June 2016, while I was still in phase 1 of my treatments, I started having weird thoughts and hallucinating. I was unable to sleep because I was afraid of my dreams. Everything I knew and believed in seemed to be crumbling under my feet. I became afraid of my shadows. After discussing at length with my wife, we decided to seek experts advice from my oncologist and our physician friend. Both of

> *"Everything I knew and believed in seemed to be crumbling under my feet. I became afraid of my shadows."*

them said it was as a result of the drugs, and that it will go away with time. They also said it might get worsened before it gets better.

This situation lasted for a few weeks. Within these periods, my prescriptions were changed. I also started attending worship fellowships and group prayer meetings. These meetings helped me tremendously to take away my thoughts and my mind from my situation, and to focus on Christ, the object of my faith. At a point, my wife called on some of our regular visitors and family friends to sing praise and worship songs anytime they visited us at home.

When you are in situations similar to these, consider some of the following. They may help you as they have helped me:

- Singing songs of praise and worship the Lord
- Praying to God for mercy and healing
- Joining others in corporate worship
- Listening to digitally recorded scriptures
- Seeking professional advice
- Talking to your doctor

*   *   *

Coping Emotionally

One of the challenges of cancer patients is loneliness. Because the treatment is long, it's almost impossible to see people that will stay with you throughout the stages. There might be times when even if they want to, the challenges in their lives may not allow this support.

Some of the critical moments when friends, well-wishers, caregivers or family members are needed include:

1. The early stages when the news is broken to the patient with the disease diagnosis. This is a moment unlike any other. It is the time when patients feel bereaved of everything. The whole world seems to collapse, and momentarily, it seems as if God has forsaken them. This is the time such questions like, "why me?", "what have I done wrong?", "where did I miss it?" and several more like these run through your mind. The patient needs the presence of trusted and mature friends and family members for encouragement, support, and advice.

I am eternally grateful to God for the people around me. Starting with my wife and co-author, what a virtuous woman she is, to Pastor Tubosun

Sowunmi who spent seven days of vigil in my house praying ceaselessly, to Alhaji Ola-Ojetola and so many other people in between. How do you ever thank such people? Thank You.

2. During the critical stages and times of admissions to the hospital when no one knows what the next moment may bring; times when the loneliness has spread to include your spouse because she (or he) has

> *"Cancer treatment does not end at the end of chemotherapy, radiation, transplant or even on the discharged day."*

become physically, emotionally and mentally exhausted and drained; times when your caregiver needs as much support as the patient.

A heartfelt appreciation and thanks to my neighbours, the good people of the Nigerian Community in Calgary, my church families, my colleagues and a host of pastors and others for their encouragements, prayers and positive thoughts.

3. At home, after you have been discharged, when the cloud has settled, and you are faced with the reality of your new life. The patient must not be left to him or herself at the culmination of the mainstream treatment.

Cancer treatment does not end at the end of chemotherapy, radiation, transplant or even on the discharge day. There are always follow-up appointments and maintenance treatments, which are equally demanding and require the support of caregivers, families, and friends.

My wife and I were never left alone. Our church families and our communities have been very magnanimous in all areas. Special appreciation and thanks go to many people for their tireless visitations – please see the *Thank You* chapter.

Lastly, the emotional effects on immediate family members are the greatest, more so, when they are also the primary caregivers. These people require as much support as the patient. In certain areas that concern both the patient and the caregiver, for example, the intimacy area, it's very advisable to seek professional help.

At the TBCC, the Multi-disciplinary OASIS[‡] [36] department has experienced and understanding professional who were always ready to guide. In addition, there are many free brochures and free seminars on how to manage sexual relationship during cancer treatments.

It is important that you discuss your situation with your oncologist or medical team.

Many thanks to Mrs. Yinka Marcus of Hope Alive Counselling Services for offering her professional services to us at no cost when we needed it most.

[‡] OASIS - Oncology and Sexuality, Intimacy and Survivorship Sexual Health Clinic

PART 2

MY EXPERIENCE

CHAPTER FOUR

MY STORY

Journey to Second Chance

Consider it all joy, my brethren, when you encounter various trials, knowing that the testing of your faith produces endurance. And let endurance have its perfect result, so that you may be perfect and complete, lacking in nothing.   James 1:2-4 (NIV)

The News!

The last week of March 2016 was also the Easter week. On Good Friday March 25th, I was able to relax my legs because it was a public holiday. However, my left hip was somehow still very painful, and in the evening, we decided to visit

67

a Chinese market for consultation with Chinese doctors. The Chinese doctor I saw prescribed acupuncture and some Chinese herbal tea. We bought the herbal tea, and I did the acupuncture immediately, and was told to come back the following Friday which was April 1st, 2016.

By the following day on Saturday 26th of March, 2016, the pain had spread to other parts of my body. I was having pains on my left shoulder

> *"That singular act and Mercy of God is about the reason I am still living today."*

and right ribs in addition to the left hip which had become more acute. By the evening, I could no longer bear the pains and at about 02:00 am on Sunday, March 27, my wife and I went to the emergency room (ER) of Foothills Medical Centre (FMC).

We were at the ER till around 17:00 (05:00 pm) on the Easter Sunday. The pains have subsided because of the palliative drugs that were given to me, but the doctors were still unable to identify or pinpoint any particular cause of my pains. Papers were prepared for my discharge, and the doctor said, "If the pains come back, you know where we are."

As we were getting up to leave, one of the doctors jokingly asked what my age was. Even though the answer was there in my file that he was holding, I replied and told him my age. The doctor continued that it is not typical for someone of my age to be having these kind of pains. He then suggested that I should go for another X-ray if I wouldn't mind!

That was the X-ray that started everything! If the X-ray were not done, I would have gone back home to continue nursing my pains until it would have probably been too late! I am eternally grateful to that doctor and, of course, to God for quickening the doctor's mind to suggest the x-ray. That singular act and Mercy of God is about the reason I am still living today.

The X-ray showed some tumour that could not be confirmed that day, and I was asked to come back the following day, for a complete CT scan.

March 30, 2016, we went back for the oncologist's report, and we had it! Multiple Myeloma!! By this time, I was already lost deep in thoughts on the potential implication of this on my life, going forward.

"You will have to start the treatment immediately," the doctor said.

"No," my wife replied. "We need time to understand and digest this information. We need to discuss with the family. Can we get a second opinion?" and many more my wife was asking the doctor.

> "The number one reason for a second opinion in cancer diagnosis is to provide clarity, and remove potential ambiguities..."

I was given three different drugs to use pending our decision on the second opinion. We later discovered that these drugs were chemo preparatory drugs.

We decided not to seek a second opinion because of a few reasons:

1. It appeared that my cancer's current stage was between stage II and stage III. Multiple myeloma only has three stages[37] and any further delay may not be advisable.

2. Most of the recommendations/advices from our friend physicians, home and abroad, suggested that we proceed with the current finding.
3. Seeking for second opinion in our area would be very challenging and expensive due to scarcity or lack of private practicing oncologists/physicians. We would have to go to a different province or country altogether.

The number one reason why people seek for a second opinion in cancer diagnosis is to provide clarity, and remove potential ambiguities from

"The need or demand for a second opinion will depend on the type of health care system that is available in your area..."

the mind of the patient on the correctness of the diagnosis. It is also to reconfirm the diagnosis and remove potential false positive. The need or demand for a second opinion will depend on the type of health care system that is available in your area (whether government sponsored, privately owned and operated, or a mixture of these).

In a mixed environment or privately owned and operated health care system, the need for the second opinion may not be over emphasized. It could mean the difference between life and death at the extreme cases.

* * *

The Treatment Phase I – Chemotherapy

In the cancer treatment world, there is a common parlance that different patients not only react to same treatment differently, but that they also show different symptoms and demonstrate diverse side effects.

I started the chemotherapy preparatory drugs on Thursday, March 31, 2016, and by the evening of the following day, I started to have hiccups. By the early hours of Sunday, April 3rd, 2016, I couldn't bear the hiccups any longer, and my wife and I headed to the ER where I was treated and discharged several hours later.

My first chemotherapy was scheduled for the first Thursday of April 2016 (07/04/2016). Everything went smoothly on the day of the Chemo, but on the second day, I started to show certain "common" side effect of one of the Chemo drugs - hiccups. Since the side effect was expected, I decided to hold on and observe for a little longer.

In the early hours of Saturday, April 9th, I could no longer curtail the situation, and we decided to head to the ER. What we thought was a simple thing turned out to be something enormous! I was admitted to Unit 32 of the Foothills Medical Centre, (FMC) and was to be retained there for the next three weeks.

* * *

Hiccups And The First Admission

We all have hiccups at some points, and in my wildest imagination, I never thought that hiccups could send someone to the hospital.

The side effect that took me to the hospital in early April was hiccups. It was so severe that I felt it was literally tearing my chest. I guessed that the potential impact of the hiccups, my physical condition, and the nearness of the impacted areas to the heart made the doctors pay quick attention to me at the ER. I was given a bed within the first hour of reaching the ER, and an Electrocardiogram (ECG) test was performed to determine the state of my heart. We were surprised to learn that there were no drugs for hiccups! Several other palliative drugs were administered, but the hiccups incessantly continued.

Within the first week of my admission, my energy was so drained that I could neither stand up nor walk. One day, I was wheeled by Mrs. Ogunleye & my wife to the McCaig centre foyer

> *"In whatever situation we may find ourselves, we are never alone."*

of the Foothills Medical Centre, and to the outside of the hall. Then it dawned on me what we take for granted when we are healthy. The freedom to move up and down and go anywhere we like, the ability to eat and drink what, where and when we like, and the power to defecate whenever we need to, have become so intimate to us that we forget how important they are.

As I was wheeled around for my chemotherapy, other medications and laboratory services, and as I spent my days in this unit, I saw patients with varying degrees of illnesses. I came across survivors and fighters like myself. I remembered that in whatever situation we may find ourselves, we are never alone. My prayer is that we may be counted among the living, the healthy and the wise – those who appreciate everything that has been given to them.

The hiccups were accompanied with severe pains and general weakness, which lingered for many following days. While the doctors were still trying to figure out how to manage my pains, a miraculous "cure" for the hiccups was found in a children's cracker biscuit that was given to us by a very good family friend and well-wisher.

Due to high volume of visitors I was having, I became so popular in the unit. Almost everyone that heard of my sickness and admission came to visit me and to wish me well.

On April 29, I was discharged from the hospital to continue the cancer treatments from home. This was the beginning of what turned out to be a one-year long intensive consultation, laboratory works, therapy, and treatments.

* * *

The Treatment Phase II – Stem Cell Transplant

Between the months of May to August, my cancer treatments went on smoothly with a weekly chemotherapy and monthly bone enhancing treatments called Zometa. In August, I began the preparations for the phase 2 of my treatments, i.e. preparation towards the stem cell transplant.

At this point, I would like to familiarize you with a part of the Tom Baker's cancer treatment procedure. Looking back, I can say that TBCC is one of the best, if not the best, in the country. TBCC has adequate resources for the physical and emotional well being of the patients and the caregivers. The nurses and the doctors, and other para-medical staff are well trained and cultured in ways that pull away stress and heaviness from the heart and the mind of the patient, at least for a time.

No stone was left unturned to diagnose the spread of cancer, particularly to potential areas or organs of the body that may be impacted or affected.

Before the commencement of my phase-2 treatments, serious clinical examinations were made of my heart, kidneys, livers, lungs, and teeth to determine their current state or baseline, as I was told. One of the advantages of these baselines, I was told, was to determine the level of changes, if any, as a result of the cancer treatment drugs, and for reversing the effects where necessary and possible.

During the first phase, the chemo was administered once weekly, and the quantity was very minimal in the order of milligram. During this phase, chemo was specifically arranged and prepared for, and the quantity was much larger.

* * *

The First Infection

Towards autologous transplanting procedure, patients are made to boost their white blood cell production by a daily injection of G-CSF drug for a whole week. Within this week, the patient is asked to watch out for any signs of fever and/or other side effects.

One morning, within the G-CSF injection week, I was scheduled for routine follow-ups, orientations, and preparations for Apheresis admission at the clinic.

Apheresis is a procedure for the collection of stem cells from the blood. That morning, during the vital signs checkup, my temperature read 39 degrees Celsius. The nurse in charge thought that it was only a spike caused by the direct exposure to the sun where I was sitting, plus the morning stress. So, I was moved to another location and asked to wait and rest a while in order to recheck the temperature. About 30 minutes later, the temperature fell below 38 degrees, and I was allowed to leave.

After the checkup and other activities for the day, we went home! What a long day!

The day had been very tiring, and I was drained; so as we got home, I went to bed immediately.

Not long after I felt asleep, I started to shiver. My wife checked my temperature and called the cancer clinic. The on-call doctor-in-charge asked us to go to the hospital immediately.

Moments later, we got to the cancer centre, and I was admitted and allotted a bed. Vitals were checked, and some palliative drugs were administered while waiting for the on-call doctor.

Then the drama started! Initially, it was an ordinary shivering, and the nurse and others around were asking me how I was feeling, etc. Then the shivering turned to rigor, shaking the whole bed, and other nurses came around to help hold me down and together. This drama lasted some minutes until I was given a drug that eventually calmed me down. After that the blood work was started to determine the cause of shivering and rigor. Thanks to Mr. & Mrs. Ofiuvwo and my wife for being around at that moment.

On the third day, I was discharged because there was no growth on the cultured blood, implying no infections could be identified.

Because no bacterial infection was detected in the blood work, it was decided that I continue with the original schedule. So, on the following

Monday, I reported for admission for the continuation of phase 2 of my treatment – the stem cell transplant stage.

The stem cell transplant process includes:

1. Administering of G-CSF – as mentioned above
2. The Apheresis procedure – stem cell collection
3. A special, high-dose chemotherapy
4. Autologous stem cell transplant

* * *

The Apheresis procedure

Before transplant can occur, stem cells are to be harvested from the bone marrow. The G-CSF was used to obtain the stem cells out of the bone marrow into the blood stream. The Apheresis process can begin, once it has been determined through blood work that sufficient stem cells are present in the blood.

Apheresis may not be a very common procedure, but it can be understood by considering the dialysis process. In dialysis, blood is passed through dialysis devices in order to separate and extract water and other components from the blood. Pure or clean blood is then passed back into the body of the patient.

In Apheresis, blood is passed through the apheresis devices to separate and extract stem cells from the blood. The blood, without stem cells, is passed into the patient's body. In summary, the apheresis devices are used to extract bone marrow (stem cells) from the blood. The stem cell extracted is subsequently used for the transplant.

In my case, the apheresis process took entire two (2) days, and it was done before my admission to the phase 2.

The Second Infection - Code 66

After we had checked in at the famous Unit 57 of the Tom Baker Cancer Centre, I was settled into a room already prepared for my overnight hydration, and other procedures towards the transplant.

Not long after I settled down, the nurses started to take my vitals while my wife stood by, watching. Then I began to shiver again, followed by rigor! My wife was trying to encourage me and calm me down, but suddenly, her voice started to fade as if she was very far off from me, and...

According to the hospital records, code 66 was called by the nurse when my eyes "drift closed", and I was "unable to follow commands to stand, sit, move my leg, etc." The ICU Outreach Team record shows that they were called because of Loss of Consciousness (LOC), and their Goals of care was "medical care and interventions including Resuscitation" followed by ICU.

I woke up or was resuscitated a few minutes later, only to find seven or eight specialist doctors and nurses around my bed – I had "passed out," and was unconscious for some moment.

The ICU doctors left after I was stabilized, and after some question and answer session. I was later told that I had an infection, and that I had to go through the blood work process. Blood was taken from the CVC, as well as, directly from my veins. In the morning, I was told that I had been infected with a strain of bacterial through my CVC central line, as the blood taken from CVC had shown some growth. Therefore, the CVC had to be removed. The same morning, the CVC was taken out.

Recovering from this infection was not going to be as quick as the first time! I was kept in the hospital for a few days, and the transplant that was supposed to start the following day was now postponed almost indefinitely, because nothing could be done until I was completely free of the infection.

* * *

The CVC & the PICC Lines

The Central Venous Catheter (CVC) & the Peripherally Inserted Central Catheter (PICC) Line

The Central Venous Catheter (CVC), generally called Central Line or CVC "is a thin, flexible tube (catheter) that is placed into the large vein above the heart, usually through a vein in the neck, chest or arm."[38]

The central line was inserted in preparation for the transplant. And now, with the central line removed, the medical team needed another way to transfer the stem cells into my body. It was agreed to use PICC Line.

A peripherally inserted central catheter (PICC), or PICC line, "is a catheter that is placed in the antecubital vein (a large vein in the inner elbow area). It is threaded through the vein into or near the right atrium of the heart."[39]

About one week after my second infection ordeal, I was scheduled for the installation of the PICC line. With the insertion of the PICC, I was, once again, back on the schedule for the stem cell transplant.

A CVC or PICC or other similar process or device is required for the transplant.

The Special Chemo

All along my treatments, there were only two occasions when I had to take a special dosage of chemo drugs.

My first special high-dosage chemotherapy was just before I started the boosting of my stem cells with the use of G-CSF injection. It was administered in August, and the objective was to inject me with a very heavy dose of cyclophosphamide, to kill as many of the cancer cells in my body as possible.

All along, from the beginning of my chemo in April to the end of July, I was on weekly Velcade drug for chemo. The Velcade drug was so effective in my case that by June, myeloma cells had reduced by more than 79%. Additionally, at the end of the special chemo of cyclophosphamide drug, the biopsy result showed no sign of myeloma, as the cancer cell were too negligible to count.

This is usually the end of multiple myeloma treatment before the advent of bone marrow transplant. There are also situations where patients cannot tolerate the transplant process due to age or other circumstances. In such situation, this would mark the end of treatment. However, if the treatment were to stop at this stage, the prognosis was usually not very good as the remission is said to be a lot shorter.

The second special high-dosage chemotherapy was scheduled just before the transplant. In this chemo, a different chemotherapy drug was used. One may ask that why should one go through the additional trouble if biopsy and other indicators have shown zero cancer cell? My oncologist's response to this question was simply that transplant helps to augment the length of remission period. This assertion was corroborated by a friend who had to go through the transplant just three years after he was declared multiple myeloma free.

* * *

The Melphalan Special Chemotherapy

As mentioned above, multiple myeloma treatment without stem cell transplant has a shorter remission period for most patients. So, I was rescheduled for transplant after the infection had been cured.

A day to the transplant, I was to take a very high dosage of melphalan drug. The objective, according to my oncologist, was to kill any potential remnants of myeloma cell within my body. But melphalan has a very bad reputation because of its horrible and damaging side effects. One of the most critical and serious side effects is what it does to the mouth, oesophagus, the intestine, and the anus. To prevent this serious side effect, a patient needs to literally eat ice cubes for a minimum of six to seven hours!

The melphalan process takes about 30 minutes to complete, so the patient must be on ice cubes for about an hour before melphalan process starts, and at least six hours after it has been completely injected.

With the eating of ice cube for six hours, you would have thought the worst is over with respect to melphalan's side effect. You can never be more wrong! Ice eating only reduced the side effect!!. Prior to the use of ice cubes, it was said that patients sometimes end up at the ICU because of the melphalan's side effects.

For two weeks, after the application, I was literally on fluids only. The mouth, the throat, the intestine and the anus/rectum were so sore that eating, drinking and going to the toilet became extremely difficult, more like Herculean tasks.

The Autologous stem cell transplant

Stem cells used for the transplant can be obtained from the patient or a donor; and when it is from the patient, it is called AUTOLOGOUS. The stem cells collected through the apheresis process described earlier, are stored in the appropriate frozen condition. They were brought in, in a special device that, I suppose, was meant to ensure continued preservation and optimum condition, even when the cells have been taken out of storage. Two nurses were looking after the stem cells.

Another nurse, who was responsible for fixing me up with the tubes and connecting the PICC lines, was busy on one side of my bed. At the other side, the vital sign equipment was placed.

The whole process took less than 30 minutes, and the stem cell transplant was complete!

A few hours later, on the same day, I was asked to go home. With several different medicines, including anaesthesia drug, anti-nausea, laxative and a few others, we headed home – I was home for the Thanksgiving Weekend!

While we were at home, we were asked to watch out, mostly, for fever (temperature above 38.0

degree Celsius), and any other abnormal conditions. The first two days went by without any incidents. On the fourth day, however, we headed back to admission after we had called. And this began another serious session of more than two weeks of admission.

* * *

The Third Infection and the HPTP

One week after my transplant, my immunity was expected to go down to zero, and it complied. I had to take extra care to guard against infections. I was not allowed to go out or receive visitors, and if I needed to move around, I had to wear protection to cover my mouth and nose.

By the end of the first week, the effect of melphalan started to manifest with a sore throat, difficulties in swallowing and going to the washroom, and gross, uncomfortable feeling of pain, weakness, and tiredness.

Early one morning, the doctor walked in and told me that the PICC line must be removed, as

I have tested positive to another bacterial infection. With the removal of PICC, I returned to being poked many times every day for blood work.

For a few days, I was essentially on liquid food because of a sore throat and unsettled stomach. My wife would blend meat, *Amala, and Ewedu* (local food) together for me to drink or take like a smoothie (pure solid food). At the same time, I was on antibiotics for my infections.

About two weeks after my transplant, my immunity started to come up, and precisely 14 days after my transplant, I was discharged from the famous unit 57 of Tom Baker Cancer Centre.

I was discharged to go home, yes, but my infection was not yet cured. So, I had to be transferred to the Home Parenteral Therapy Program (HPTP) to continue with them for home care. I was with HPTP for one month, and during this period, I had to carry self-medication IV machine 24 hrs. per day. Within that period, the home nurses visited me between four to six times to dress my IV and change the machine battery. On November 20th, I was fully and finally discharged – Praise God!

* * *

Maintenance Medication

Every cancer that has been successfully treated has a remission period. The remission period depends on several factors, including if there is a maintenance requirement after the treatment or not, the type or nature of cancer, and the patient, among other factors.

The remission period for multiple myeloma also varies according to these factors.

Maintenance of patient to prolong the remission period includes the administration of chemotherapy after the patient has been discharged, and the use of certain remission drugs, among others. Like during the treatment phases, chemoteraphy may be in the form of tablets, injections, IV, or a combination of these.

Because of the serious side effects of the chemotherapy, my maintenance did not include chemotherapy. I was put on some remission drugs, which are again, not without their own side effects. In fact, in the beginning, I had to suspend the drug and later resumed with a lower dosage.

Within the past one year, I have come across different people (fighters and survivors) who are at different stages of their myeloma treatment.

Generally speaking, and with the advancement in technology, there is an increase in optimism with myeloma, and survivors are now living much longer.[40] The average remission period for multiple myeloma can be as long as nine years, according to my oncologist, who also said he has a patient who has not come back since the late 1990s. Recently we met a family with a patient who has been on remission for over 18 years and still going strong.

* * *

Phase III - Kyphoplasty

One of the reasons why cancer is such a nasty disease is that it destroys everything in it's path. Even when the cancer cells themselves have been eradicated, the damage they have caused will more likely remain behind.

Multiple Myeloma is a cancer of the plasma cells or in other words, cancer of bones and blood (bone marrow). In my case, myeloma compromised my bones (spine) and bone marrow. The solution to bone marrow was a stem cell transplant in addition to the chemo treatements. In October 2016, I had a successful autologous stem cell transplant. But some parts of my bones (spine) were also compromised! It occurred to me that my doctors were addressing my situation one after another.

By January 2017, I started feeling the effect of my weakened spine; I could not sit properly, or for long, I could not stand up straight. I was always in pain and could not walk properly. Some sections of my spine were severely damaged to the extent that it may collapse or break with a minimal accident or fall.

With this knowledge, my oncologist prescribed a kyphoplasty[41] surgery – a minimally invasive surgery used to treat a spinal compression fracture. This was supposed to be a few hour surgery, and my son took the day off to come to Calgary. The three of us, including my wife, went to the South Health Campus for the surgery. The doctor is one of the best, we were told; however, during the surgery, there were complications, and the surgeon said that was the first time that it would happen.

Some "cement" particles went into parts of my lungs, and a pulmonary doctor was called. The pulmonary doctor also said, it was very rare, and had to summon his colleagues for advice.

I was supposed to be discharged the same day, but had to be retained in the hospital and monitored the next two days.

To God be the glory, after all the necessary tests, scans and x-rays, nothing to be worried about was found; I could breathe and eat well.

Six weeks later, other pulmonary tests and CT Scans were performed and Praise God; I am ok.

PART 3

FROM THE EYE OF THE SPOUSE – THE CAREGIVER

CHAPTER FIVE

Cancer Treatments and the Art of

CAREGIVING

Let us not lose heart in doing good, for in due time we will reap if we do not grow weary. So then, while we have opportunity, let us do good to all people, and especially to those who are of the household of the faith. Galatians 6:9-10 (NIV)

Who Is A Caregiver?

To my understanding, a caregiver is a person who provides help and supports a sick person. While some caregivers are being paid, some are not paid. The unpaid caregivers and volunteers are usually family members, relatives or spouses. In my case, I am the spouse.

Caregivers provide a variety of support to different people at various times, including spouse, children, partner, parent or a young adult. Their role is very crucial and cardinal in the patient's care because they ensure both emotional and physical well-being of the patient.

It all started in January 2016, after he returned from work. He said he had pulled his ribs while on the "job training" at work; it seemed like a normal pain, but as time went on, it became unbearable! He did all the necessary tests, including comprehensive medical checkup. The yearly cancer screen also came out negative, and we received a letter from the government stating that he's cancer free! But the pain refused to go!

The Easter Weekend was spent at the emergency, and that's where a tumour was discovered on the side where he had complained in January.

*   *   *

On the fateful day of March 27th, 2016; we had Easter Egg Hunt at BP Church, where I volunteered. Later that day, I attended an award program at another event. As the evening progressed, I had a hunch to go home early and therefore, requested that my award be brought forward; I received the award and left. Thanks to Mozia Women's Network for their understanding.

That night, he could not sleep very well due to pain. He woke me up around 2:00 am with excruciating pain, and he said, "My dear, we have to go to the emergency." We all know that when a man requests to go to the emergency, it must mean that the situation is at it's worse. We set out around 2:00am in the early morning of the Easter Sunday. There we were until around 5:00pm; with all the tests conducted that day, nothing substantial was found.

We were already being discharged when a "God sent doctor" decided to order an X-ray they would normally do for people of ages 60 years and above; this was the scan that opened the can of worms.

Thank goodness, the X-ray was ordered, and we were immediately asked to report for a comprehensive CT scan the following day, on Easter Monday. His CT scan was placed on priority, the result was released the same day, and we pensively waited for the doctor's interpretation at the emergency. At some point, I saw the doctors calling themselves and reviewing his file on the computer, and heard them talking about an oncologist, hematologist, and other things. Outwardly, I stayed calm and strong, but had a million questions running through my head and my mind; I was like, "I hope that's not for us."

After some time, the doctor came in and started to talk softly. When I heard Myeloma for the first time, I didn't know that it was cancer, until he

> *"Why do you want a second opinion, ...it may be late by the time you get the result."*

said it is a cancer of the Plasma Cells. This was the first time I heard the term Myeloma; we have always heard about other types of cancer as prostate, lung, cervical, breast, and a host of others. I didn't know what questions to ask; I paused and started to pray and sing to God inside. Not too long, my energy came back, and I started asking all sorts of questions. I am sure the doctor was tired of my questions, although, he did try to answer each one of them to the best of his knowledge.

We were referred to the oncologist/haematologist, and the emergency doctor said a biopsy would be conducted by the haematologist, but I had no idea what to expect.

When we met the haematologist, the lady doctor started to talk softly, and I said to her, "Please speak up so I can hear you clearly;" I also said to her… "Please tell me exactly what is going on." She paused, I'm sure she didn't know how I would react. Then she said, "Mr. Oladele has Multiple Myeloma, a cancer of the Plasma Cells." That confirmed the emergency doctor's assertion, and opened an additional array of questions, and I said I would like to have a second opinion. She tried to convince me not to have it, but all she said fell on deaf ears.

Then another very soft spoken doctor came in and asked, "Why do you want a second opinion and that even if you do, it may be late by the time you get the result." It was then that I paused! I guessed since they have seen the CT scan and all the blood work, they knew they had to do something immediately.

After the consultation, we were asked to go to another room. At that point, I wasn't aware that it was for the biopsy because my husband could not walk properly. I thought he was going to be properly examined on the bed, until I saw different gadgets! The biopsy was supposed to take about 10-15 minutes, but due to some complications, it took more than the stipulated time.

Although, they were supposed to use just one pack of the equipment, by the time they were done, about four packs were used. It had been an excruciatingly painful experience for him!

At that time, my mind was filled with a million questions, and there was no one to answer them except God. Even though he was in serious pain, the doctor still had to perform the biopsy, which

> *"...when you are around a sick person, you have to conduct yourself with a smile even when you are tired and drained."*

in itself, was very painful. I sat there facing the wall, couldn't pray, couldn't sing, couldn't do anything; I was just there. Then I summed up the courage to ask the father in heaven for guidance, direction, and what to do. How do I handle this? Who do I call? What next Lord? And so many other questions screamed inside my head.

Then I said, "Lord, please have mercy" and looked up at the ceiling, I needed to talk to someone, and I asked God for help. I needed someone who would be able to help, provide good guidance, and be of value; not someone who will start to cry or to sympathize. Then a name came to mind, and I sent a long SMS message to Dr. Sam Oluwadairo, one of our family friends and a doctor at the hospital. The Lord used him for us tremendously; only God will reward him and his family. We cannot thank them enough.

It is essential to know that when a spouse/ partner is diagnosed with a malignancy, it takes a toll on the other partner to provide all the necessary care. I had no idea what to expect, or how long/far the journey will be, and concurrently, I was devastated with the diagnosis. I have been very vocal about the importance of family, friends, and association, especially when people don't want to be associated with the people around them. Our native country is very far, and if we don't come together, sometimes it hurts. I thank God for the

Nigerians in Calgary, our church members, and our friends.

Since his mobility was impaired, I had to be the driver, and perform daily and weekly routine and tasks including, booking appointments, preparing meals, house cleaning, bill payment and driving to and from appointments, dealing with doctors and nurses, psychosocial doctors, nutritionist, social workers, pharmacists, and so on.

It can be stressful sometimes because, if you have been living with someone who does everything by himself and suddenly, the person cannot eat, walk, stand, dress, and shower – these activities squarely fall as a burden on your

> *"It is when you have a life and are not laying on the sickbed that you can think of work, business or money."*

shoulders! I had to read and understand the medications carefully. Keep a consistent tab to know the medication that is working well and one that needs improvement. I had to quickly learn that when you are around a sick person, you have to conduct yourself with a smile even when you are tired and drained. This is important because, you cannot show sad face or emotions around a sick person. My saving grace is that I always smile, laughter comes to me naturally, and I thank God for His grace.

When the treatment started, I had to put my career and business on hold in order to devote all my time and attention to help my husband get well. I lost the majority of my clients, spent all the money, and my business suffered, but I believed that where there is life, there is hope; and I believe that God will restore all that we lost, even better! And I always say that "It is when you have a life and are not laying on the sickbed that you can think of work, business or money."

> *"Things that my husband used to do that I would normally just ask how they are going - now become mine!"*

This was a very difficult period in our lives; but as difficult as it was, I did not keep quiet. Since I could not pray, I asked for prayers from all the people of God around us in Canada, the USA and around the world; our church family, our friends, and relatives.

Having lost my mother to breast cancer in 1995, I knew that the journey will require the grace of God. She became very ill in 1975 and had mastectomy in 1985. Though she was given six months to live in 1986, with the grace of God and prayers of the faithfuls, her life was spared till 1995.

My nature of business enabled me to work with pastors and churches; when the challenges came, the majority of pastors in Calgary visited our house and hospital, and everyone I came across. One of our pastor friends, who is also a brother, spent seven days of vigil in our house with the anointed rug and oil from the General Overseer. He came every night to pray with us, sometimes, even when we were too tired to join him. It is only God, who is the rewarder of good, that will reward him. Thank you very much Pastor Tubosun Sowunmi.

Our house became a fellowship centre, prayers were offered at various times, and I am deeply appreciative of everyone. Some people could not come physically, but called and prayed over the phone, social media, WhatsApp, SMS, email and so on. God moved in supernatural ways!

As I wrote earlier, when my husband was diagnosed with Multiple Myeloma, at first, I didn't understand what it was; I researched and read about it a few times on my phone, and it still didn't make any sense. Not because I didn't understand the explanation, but because I was simply looking at the phone without applying my mind, and everything seemed blank. I was just looking as if nothing was written on the pages. Everything the doctor was saying sounded Greek or an unknown language. It was like I didn't hear what they were saying.

"God will not allow two people's load to become one person's."

Because some of us are healthy, we take for granted things that come to us naturally. Glory be to God, for granting us health. I found that things that my husband used to do that I would normally just ask how they are going - now became mine, like laundry, taking out the garbage, car maintenance, and other chores. There is an adage in my place that says, "God will not allow two people's load to become one person's."

* * *

As no one prepares for things like this, I had to learn on the go; below are some of what I learnt:

1. Mobility: when the pain became worse, and he could not walk properly or perform Activities of Daily Living (ADLs), I had to look for a walking-cane so that he could use it to support himself. Sometimes, climbing the stairs would be tough, and hence, we had to move to the main floor for easy movement.

2. Home Maintenance: these included both the outside and inside of the home:

    a. **Snow Removal**: it's like we had lots of snow in 2016, and it was so difficult initially. The fact that our son does not live in the city made it more difficult. However, he was able to help anytime he came to visit. My brother-in-law also was a great help, and at some point, we had to engage a snow clearing company to perform the snow removal for us.

b. **Lawn Cutting**: this was no problem in spring/summer 2016 because we had already engaged the services of a lawn mowing company. However, in 2017, our neighbor's sons, John and Joseph Ogunleye were able to clear our snow and mown the lawn – thank you boys!

c. **Plumbing & Heating**: whenever things are needed to be repaired at home, thank God for Odion Oshodin who always makes himself available. We can call on him at any time and, gratitude to his wife, Linda, for allowing him to come whenever we require his help.

d. **General House Cleaning**: when the news was broken to us, everything became so bleak and dirty. I didn't care how messy the house was, and I said to myself, "Whoever comes to my house and does not like it, can leave." Housekeeping was not my priority at that time. In fact, house cleaning was the last thing on my mind. However, as time progressed, I was able to call on our house cleaner to take care of the house.

3. The caregiver also needs to be cared for: I noticed that with the number of people that trooped to the house and hospital, most people did not ask how I was faring. Some days, my energy would be so low that I simply needed someone who would talk to me; but instead, people would call and ask how my husband was doing.

However, there were indeed a few people who would engage me in a long talk, to ensure I do not fall asleep, either when I would be going home from the hospital, or in the morning. I remember one day, I was in the hospital's parking lot, and was having negative thoughts. One of my friends Mrs. Bola Esan, phoned me, she was Godsend, she started to talk mainly, how I have been feeling that day and that I should please take care of myself, and she gave me one scenario which woke me up.

My prayer group also helped – the Prayer Chain at BP Church and Princess of the Kings Prayer group! They prayed daily until my husband was discharged from the hospital in late April.

* * *

Breaking the news to the family

Breaking the news to the family was not easy; my sister and my brother-in-law had been with us for about six months, my sister left in January while my brother-in-law left early March. Although, they were aware of his shoulder pain, but no one knew the cause. I didn't know how to tell them because I was emotional myself, it was like breaking bad news; I love to be a good news bearer!

This situation fell on my shoulder as my husband was fighting within himself and asking God why; I don't see him calling and informing his siblings. Earlier in the week, I had messaged my brother-in-law to continue to pray because the pain was becoming unbearable. So, I called and informed him being the most senior, and he would disseminate to others. Since almost all our siblings are pastors, prayers were said at different times, including fasting.

My siblings and my friend - Mrs. Remi Oyefeso were always calling, praying and checking up on me. Canada is too far; we live in a place where people cannot just decide to visit anyhow as it takes about 22 hours to get to Canada from Nigeria. Even if they wanted to come, the Canadian Embassy in Nigeria were not helpful; visa applications were denied to most of our siblings, so I was lonely until my brother-in-law was able to come.

To our newly married son and his wife, they had just given us the good news of their family expansion. At first, we didn't know how to tell/break the news to them. How could this be? Not now! How do I tell them or what do I say? I didn't want to upset either of them knowing his wife's condition; so we prayed for God's guidance and direction. Then we called them to come home on the weekend; even though they both asked lots of questions, we decided not to tell them anything since they live out of town, and driving 2.5 hours to the city.

It was very shocking when the news was broken to them; they were in disbelieve and like me, after a while, Lekan asked, "What's next thing?" How do we proceed, etc., and other questions.

During the course of the treatment, we got a big binder of information about the stem cell transplant, which detailed the process and challenges. I gave the binder to Lekan, to go through and revert. There is one of the topics that talked about "the patient may die during the process." I noticed he got emotional and was asking questions; unfortunately, I was unable to provide answers.

In July 2016, four of us (myself, my husband, Lekan and Zandra) met with the oncologist and the Bone Marrow Transplant (BMT) staff to go over the stem cell transplant process; it was too much information to process at once. We all asked different questions, and they answered them appropriately.

Our family has been very supportive, despite Zandra' s condition, she will make various types of food and send them through Lekan; we are blessed to have her!

Mrs. Ada Ocholi (Zandra' s mum), she is not a mother-in-law, she is a "sister from another mother". We became one family, I can call on her at any time, and despite her tight schedule, she will bring the food or anything I asked for if it's within her power. One day, I wanted *akara* (beans cake), I just called her, she brought the whole items to my house, and we made the akara together; it was fun!!! That taught me that you can still have fun in the middle of a situation.

> *"We are all caregivers at some point in our lives!"*

Lesson Learnt

We are all caregivers at some point in our lives, either we care for our children, family members, ageing parents, and the list goes on. We often forget to observe some of the lessons learnt so we can apply it to other situations. We tend to deal with the situation as they arise, and that's ok, because each situation is unique and the way we deal with them are different.

During this process, I had a few things that I observed and considered as common to situations:

1. **Positive Attitude:** As I said earlier, smile and laughter come to me naturally; this really helped me. Not that I was happy with the news or the situation, but I wasn't going to start crying and burst into laughter. Attitudes matter most, especially when you're sitting with someone that is being diagnosed, or someone that cannot eat or drink. There is a hymn that we used to sing when I was in choir and still resonate with me, although I know the *Yoruba* version very well, it says:

"Weeping will not save me;
Though my face was bathed in tears,
That could not allay my fears,

Could not wash the sins of years;
Weeping will not save me.

Chorus:
Jesus bled and died for me;
Jesus suffered on the tree;
Jesus waits to make me free;
He alone can save me!

2
Working will not save me;
Purest deeds that I can do
Holiest thoughts and feelings too,
Cannot form my soul anew;
Working will not save me.
3
Waiting will not save me;
Helpless, guilty, lost I lie;
In my ear is mercy's cry;
If I wait, I can but die;
Waiting will not save me.

4
Faith in Christ will save me;
Trust in Him, the risen One,
Trust the work that He has done;
To His arms I now may run;
Faith in Christ will save me."

So, I knew that weeping or wailing would not solve this problem. I am the type that does not dwell in the past; I want to move forward. When there is a problem, I like to know the solution.

115

When the lady doctor was telling us that they had reviewed the CT scan to find a Myeloma; even though I was sad, still, I was smiling. She was just looking at me, and I told her, "This is just me" before I started to ask questions.

"Consider it pure joy, my brothers and sisters, whenever you face trials of many kinds, because you know that the testing of your faith produces perseverance" James 1:2-3

2. **Self-Care:** Take care of yourself, while helping a patient to get well, you as a caregiver need to keep a tab on your medical check-up, rest, eat, look good, etc. One day, I was so tired, I picked up a phone and called a massage and acupuncture place. It felt so good! Don't neglect yourself and don't forget yourself – take care of yourself. Sometimes, the caregivers get sick while taking care of the sick because they usually neglect themselves; this was always in my mind, and I make sure that I visited our family doctor often, perform my yearly medical check-up, and make sure that the situation is not pulling me down.

3. **De-Stressed**: Caregiving is not an easy task, and can be stressful sometimes. So, you need to release tension and de-stress at some point. You can de-stress through any of the following ways: praying, exercises, Zumba, dancing, singing, group activities, cooking, massage, acupuncture and a host

> *"Cast your burdens unto Jesus for He cares for you..."*

of others. As a caregiver, you need to know your de-stressors, and remember to take it up. For me, singing helped, praise and worship, bible verses – sometimes, I would not remember where they are, but I can say for example: Cast your burdens unto Jesus for He cares for you... this is a bible verse and a song. Other songs and hymns like: Praise my soul the king of heaven, my faith looks up to thee, it is well with my soul...; Psalms 23, 35, 91, 121 were in my mouth, even though in my language.

4. **Sleep:** Monitoring the patient forms the primary aim and function of the job. It is sometimes, difficult to get good sleep, especially when your patient needs

117

medication in the midnight and the early hours of the day. One needs to catch-up with sleep so that the caregiver is neither sick nor sleepwalking. As we all know that lack of sleep leads to sickness, a sick caregiver cannot take care of the patient. We just need to nap at intervals, especially when medication has to be taken every four or six hours; one can sleep in-between. However, there are other things to be done around the house.

5. **Rest:** Often, we compare sleep to rest... I have heard some of my friends called and said, "please try and relax" and I would say to myself if I rest, who will do this and that... I was wrong! Resting is not sleeping. Resting enables your body to be refreshed and restored. Psalm 23:3 says "He renews my soul." When our body is well rested, it will improve our state of mind, mental, physical and spiritual. During his hospital admission in April, I go home at night to get some rest, and during that period, I usually have questions for the doctors the next day.

6. **Finance:** Put your finances in order. Planning and organizing day-to-day spending can be very important. Since the diagnosis was sudden, we didn't have time to re-organize our finances. We were just spending; I didn't care how much, I just wanted my husband to be well. Even though some of the drugs were covered by the Tom Baker Cancer Centre and company insurance, we still spent a lot of money in non-insurance covered prescription drugs and other items.

"Whatever you are going through, know that someone has been there, some people are there right now, and some will still be there."

At some point, we needed new dishes, cutleries, change his clothes, daily food, manage the air quality, and a host of others. Gas/fueling the car and parking at the hospital were not cheap, and all these costs added up to a substantial amount of money. Money is very essential in dealing with the sickness; no matter how much you have, you need more money.

Some may be wondering why we needed to get new items at home, for example, as the treatment progresses, he lost some weight. Hence, we had to change his wardrobe. To guard against infections due to his low immunity, his dishes, cups, cutleries and toileteries had to be changed, and a host of other things.

7. **Ask for Help:** I thought I could handle certain things by myself; but one day, a friend called and said, "You are not alone," that statement made me reach out more. Remember, whatever you are going through, know that someone has been there, some people are there right now, and some will still be there. You may not know the people, but there are thousands or millions of people having similar feelings or situation like you now. Do not keep it to yourself; ask for help whenever the need arises. For example, if you cannot cook, ask a friend to bring you food or if you cannot drive to appointments, ask a friend or call the transportation department at the hospital

The week he was diagnosed, we didn't eat very well; I tried to cook one night, it was so salty. We could not eat and had to sleep like that – this was because of the state of mind. The next day, we were sitting in our family doctor's office thinking that we'll go and get food after, when a friend sent me a message saying, "I lost my job this week." Instead of empathizing with her, I replied, "Please bring me some food; I'll be home in about an hour." I sent the same message to my neighbour as well. I'm sure they'll be thinking - before she can ask for food, something must be fishing. They did not even ask me why or what's going on. By the evening,

> "Cancer itself, is an adversary and getting into depression makes it a lot worse."

my house was full of all kinds of foods; and since then, different people have called to ask what they can do or how they can help.

Something that touched us was on 2016 Thanksgiving Weekend; we had turkey, but too tired to prepare it, and we had few family friends that visited us. I guess Mr. Ogunsola and his wife realized how tired we were and noticed no sign of turkey or festivity; the following day, they dropped off a ready to eat "Big-Turkey" for us. This made us very emotional, and decided that every year, as long as God give us breath, we will reciprocate same to some families going through tough time in the community.

8. **Ask Questions**: there are no "stupid questions." I asked questions every step of the way because I needed clarifications with medications. I would ask, "What does this do? What are the effects or implications? The doctors and care team will definitely answer and explain to your satisfaction. Even the Bible says, "Ask, and you will receive." Questions help in changing medications because if they tell you the benefits and dangers of the drugs, you can say, "Oh, I think he felt this way yesterday or in the night," and they may conclude the drug will not benefit him and thereby, change or modify it.

9. **Be Alert:** Caregiver is the lifeline of the patient. Being alert always can save the life of the patient. For example, on the night of the stem cell transplant, I noticed he was shaking, and I thought it was just cold. When I called the doctor, he told us where to go immediately. That night was not funny because it was a real infection, and what I thought was just shivering, they call it "rigor" and this happened twice. The second time, some of the ICU doctors were summoned.

Part of my alertness was to know the amount of water/fluid, food consumed in per day and quantity; watch his food; check temperature, check blood pressure, and a host of other things. For example, if the temperature is over certain degrees, we need to call the clinic, and this happened a few times.

10. **What If?:** A caregiver needs to be courageous because your courage gives strength to the sick person. Although, I was down and drained myself, especially when the fear of finances would come into my mind such as, how do we pay for the mortgage and bills. I had so many "what ifs". What if his income seizes, what if the insurance stop paying both short term and long term benefits, what if we cannot afford the drugs, what if the inevitable happens, etc. As a self-employed, I didn't think I could leverage the government support, it never crossed my mind. However, I later found out that there's not much funding for the caregivers, unless you are at the rock bottom - which our God did not allow to happen. He supplied our needs and took away my fears.

Through this journey, I learnt that Cancer itself, is an adversary and getting into depression makes it a lot worse. It can lead to another sickness if care is not taken, and the doctors will continue to prescribe drugs based on your explanation. Here, the caregiver will be able to know how often, the problem occur and if it requires medication or not.

Providing adequate and tender loving care to a person diagnosed with cancer is quite challenging. The sad truth is that cancer patients may go through a lot of emotional struggles during the entire course of the disease process; this is what makes it difficult for caregivers to get help through every stage of the battle.

* * *

I could not have gone through the process without God's help and sustenance, according to Psalm 55:22:

"Cast your cares on the LORD, and he will sustain you; he will never let the righteous be shaken."

Throughout this journey, I read many scriptures about cancer and healing, and whenever I get back from the hospital, I will replace or put his name in the scriptures. I always say and journalled, "I know my redeemer liveth." Some of the scriptures include:

1) *Psalm 23:4 Yea, though I walk through the valley of the shadow of death, I will fear no evil: for thou art with me; thy rod and thy staff they comfort me.*

2) *Jeremiah 30:17 For I will restore health unto thee, and I will heal thee of thy wounds, saith the LORD; ...*

3) *Isaiah 41:10 Fear thou not; for I am with thee: be not dismayed; for I am thy God: I will strengthen thee; yea, I will help thee; yea, I will uphold thee with the right hand of my righteousness.*

4) *Psalms 118:17 I shall not die, but live, and declare the works of the LORD.*

5) *Psalms 34:19 Many are the afflictions of the righteous: but the LORD delivereth him out of them all.*

6) *John 10:10 The thief cometh not, but for to steal, and to kill, and to destroy: I come that they might have life and that they might have it more abundantly.*

7) *Jeremiah 17:14 Heal me, O LORD, and I shall be healed;Save me, and I shall be saved,for You are my praise.*

8) *1 Peter 2:24 Who Himself bore our sins in His own body on the tree, that we, having died to sins, might live for righteousness - by whose stripes you were healed.*

9) *3 John 1:2 Beloved, I wish above all things that thou mayest prosper and be in health, even as thy soul prospereth.*

10) *Psalm 103:1-5*
   Bless the Lord, O my soul;
   And all that is within me, bless His holy name!
   [2] Bless the Lord, O my soul,
   And forget not all His benefits:
   [3] Who forgives all your iniquities,
   Who heals all your diseases,
   [4] Who redeems your life from destruction,
   Who crowns you with lovingkindness and tender mercies,
   [5] Who satisfies your mouth with good things,
   So that your youth is renewed like the eagle's.

* * *

Good News

The news about us becoming grandparents came around the same period of the diagnosis. I now had to take care of two people. The good thing is that Mrs. Ocholi our mother-in-law lives in the city; so it was not stressful. Also, our son is a very good cook, and the pressure of cooking was reduced. Our granddaughter's birth brought life and light into our family. We are very grateful for His faithfulness.

Zoë, you brought life into the family! We went from sorry to congratulations, and people no longer dwell in greeting us about the disease, but "how's your grand-daughter." We pray God's blessings, grace, and favour to be upon you every day of your life continually, and you will grow in the grace of God. You will continue to shine according to Isaiah 60: *"Arise, shine, for your light has come, and the glory of the LORD rises upon you."*

* * *

CONCLUSION

*From now on, let no one cause me trouble, for I bear on
my body the marks of Christ. Galatians 6:17 (NIV)*

Cancer is a very dangerous disease that affects
both the young and old, male and female. We
believe that if the disease is detected and
diagnosed early enough before metastasis,
there are chances for different types of
treatments, and prognosis can even be longer.
God is the healer and the great physician; we
thank God for His power of healing in our lives.

As Christians, we believe in the power of prayer
- our God is the healer of any manner of

sickness or affliction, whether it is physical, spiritual, mental, financial or emotional. We all need the healing power of God in our lives, no matter the situations, our God is good!

"For I will restore health unto thee, and I will heal thee of thy wounds, saith the LORD;" Jeremiah 30 :17 (kjv)

Technology changes every day; research into drugs and treatment to all kinds of sickness is also on the go. For myeloma, new research and treatment is being discovered daily and hopefully in no distant future, it will become a chronic and curable disease.

Presently, the chemotherapy drugs are live safers but they are not *intelligent*; they are indiscriminate and crude, they kill all cells on their path regardless of whether the cells are normal and healthy, or infected and diseased. In the future, we will have intelligent chemo drugs that will selectively target only the diseased cells. We hope that the future will not be too long or too far away.

One of the goals of writing this book is to create awareness and to educate other survivors, patients, family and community members about the disease, the risk factors and the need for taking preventive measures, and for people to donate towards cancer research and development, and most importantly, that OUR GOD IS THE GREAT PHYSICIAN.

We will achieve these by organizing seminars, workshops and by visiting different associations, churches, and communities to encourage and let people facing similar challenges know that they are not alone. While technology is on the verge of breakthrough, our God is still in the business of doing miracle, and we can heal together while sharing.

THE GRACE OF GOD!

THANK YOU

And the prayer offered in faith will make the sick person well; the Lord will raise them up. If they have sinned, they will be forgiven. James 5:15 (NIV)

Putting together this chapter made us realized the simple truth that it is impossible to know everyone who has been involved in my journey to victory. Many people have been involved in corporate prayers where prayer points were raised for people they do not know, and yet they prayed. Many people have prayed for us from the altar of God in their hearts, homes and places of worship. We may never know many of you, but God knows you. My prayer is that God reward you in multiple folds of what you have done for me and my family.

We sincerely apologized if your name has been omitted in the following pages. It is NOT intensional. The important thing is that the Great Healer, our God, knows your name and He will perfect your situation in Jesus Name.

* * *

On March 29, 2016, my wife called some of our friends to inform them of my new medical situation. Alhaji Azeez Ola-Ojetola and Alhaji Muideen Adeyemi came to our house around 11:00 pm to offer special prayers that lasted well into the night. They continued to pray and about two months later after I was discharged from my first round of admission, the Alhajis came back for another round of night prayers. This time they were accompanied by Alhaji Tunde Lawal. I am very grateful for your supports and prayers and thanks to you and the members of the Nigerian Canadian Muslims Congregation, Calgary.

On Thursday, March 31, 2016, Dr. Ogunnariwo (Dr. O.) was one of the first people to come into our house to empathize with us. When he learnt that we were thinking of a second opinion, he was very furious and disturbed. It was like he knew what may happen if we delayed in starting the chemotherapy treatment. Dr. O is one of the elders in our community. He stood with us like a father, and remained a dependable elder till the end of my treatments, and even until now.

Mr. Daniel & Mrs. Mariam Ofiuvwo, Mrs. Rachael Oguntuase, and Mr. & Mrs. Ogunleye my closest neighbors and friends, are "secondary" caregivers. Because of you, we were never lonely or without food. Thank you, so much dear neighbors and friends. With you, God has accomplished so much in my treatment and in my life, and I could not imagine what it would have been like without you.

Mr. & Mrs. Michael Odion Oshodin thank you for always being there for us; you always make sure that the house is well kept, take out the garbage and repair anything that needs to be fixed around the house.

Mr. & Mrs. Johnson & Mary Atole, Mr. & Mrs. Deji & Oluchin Atika, Grandma Nnena Oji, Mr. & Mrs. Dare & Temi Kolawole, thank you for always standing with my family. Thank you for your provisions and for your prayers.

Chief (Dr.) Sam and Chief (Mrs.) Regina Oluwadairo - Where do I start with these two great and humble servants of the community? It's becoming difficult to find anyone within the community who has not been touched by this couple. Dr. Oluwadairo was the first person my wife called on Wednesday after the Oncologist confirmed my situation. Since then, they have never abandoned us. Being a medical doctor, he was one of our technical advisers, walking with us all along the way. De-Chosen, thank you for all your supports and provisions, God will continue to bless you abundantly.

*   *   *

The Admissions, Chemotherapy and Transplant

On Friday, April 1, 2016, Pastor Ademola Farinu who was coming to Calgary from Victoria for a weekend of a special church event came straight to our house with his hosts, Pastor Leke Kelani, after he received a text message from my wife about my diagnosis. He came back again with his wife, Pastor (Mrs.) Ihuoma Farinu and Pastor Bunmi Owolabi the following day. Pastor Farinu and these other men of God visited us many other times, and continued to pray for my healing and recovery. Thank you so much for your cares, love and prayers.

Saturday, April 2, 2017, was a very busy day for us. Pastor Tim Abi-Abiola, Pastor Ben & Pastor (Mrs.) Dee Adekugbe were some of the pastors that came to our house to pray with us. Later in the week, Pastor John Adeyemi was brought in by Pastor Abiola to pray for me. Thank you so much for your continuous prayers. God who is the greatest rewarder will reward all of you.

Pastor Tubosun & Pastor (Mrs.) Moni Sowunmi – My wife had been in contact with Pastor Sowunmi since the Easter Sunday when we went to the Emergency Centre. Pastor Sowunmi and his wife have been praying for us, but on Sunday, April 3, 2016, Pastor Sowunmi came to our house at around 11:30pm to start a seven-day night vigil of prayer and worship in my home. This act of love and support was over and above my expectations. You wonder what a height of sacrifice and selflessness this was. I pray God every moment to reward you accordingly. Thank you, my friend and pastor.

Mr. & Mrs. Ocholi, my dearest in-laws, thank you for your moral, material and spiritual supports throughout my time of trial; we appreciate you, God will continue to bless you abundantly.

Mrs. Ojekale, Mr. Derin & Mrs. Moji Taiwo, Mr. Lanre & Dr. (Mrs.) Adesola Omotayo, Mr. & Mrs. Peter & Juliet Okeke, Elshadai, Mr. Ehi & Mrs. Grace Aihomu, Princess of the King's prayer group, Holy Ghost Encounter prayer group, and many others too numerous to mention, thank you so much for your prayers, supports and provisions.

After the night vigil with Pastor Sowunmi on Friday, April 8, I went to sleep in the adjourning room since I could no longer climb the stairs to go to our room. I had a very remarkable dream and shortly after my hiccup returned, and we headed back to the Emergency. This was now the second week of the start of my ordeal and many other friends, and members of our communities had been informed.

It is practically impossible to name everyone that was praying for me, came to visit and or brought food, fruits or other items. Thank you so much to everybody. May God Almighty reward you all.

Mr. & Dr. (Mrs.) Oladosu came to the emergency the moment they heard and would not leave until I was taken to a room later on that day. They continued to visit me at home with material and spiritual support; we cannot thank you enough!

Dr. & Mrs. Marcus are uncle and aunt of repute. I believe that God placed you in our lives for reasons that are yet to be fully manifested. You were always there, providing professional counselling service, holding us materially and spiritually. We really enjoyed the *Eko, efo, gbegiri* among other food items you brought to the hospital and home. God will reward your labour of love.

Pastor Noral Woodburn (Cross-Cultural Pastor) who visited me at the hospital and at home many times, Pastor Mark Williams (Lead Pastor), Pastor Brandon Sarney (Associate Pastor), the pastoral team, Men and Women Fellowships, and the entire members of the Beddington Pentecostal (BP Church) thank you for your faithful prayers and support. Indeed, the fervent prayers of the righteous avails much. (Jm 6:16b KJV). To all the families who brought us food and other supports every week, God will bless you abundantly.

Chief & Chief (Mrs.) Akanni and Engr. Sola Owoputi (from the USA), your assistance and words of encouragement, will never be forgotten. Mr. Owoputi who is also a survivor was flown in by Chief Akanni to show me practical evidence of multiple myeloma survivor and to lift my spirit when I needed it most. That was one of a kind act of love and support. At your dark hours, you will not be lonely. God will lift you up and shine light into your lives.

Mr. & Mrs. Sina Akinsanya, thank you. Where do I start, what do I say and how do I thank you? It is hard to admit that during my admissions, I always looked forward to the early morning visit of Mrs. Sola Akinsanya. She is one of our community's quiet ambassadors at the FMC. God will reward your labour of love.

Mr. & Mrs. Peter & Julie Oganwu visited me many times, even when it was apparently inconvenient for them. Throughout the periods, they never showed any indications that their loved one was also going through a similar ordeal. These two are true leaders of the community. Thank you.

Mr. & Mrs. Latilo have been with me from the beginning. Glory be to God for your "miracle" cookies! Thank you so much for your supports, provisions and your prayers, and visit with grandma.

Mr. & Mrs. Tope & Bola Esan - How can I repay Flavors Restaurant? She practically became my food supplier even when I don't ask. Some people introduced us to SourSop; before you know it, Mrs. Bola Esan has gone to various places to order the fresh leaf and the frozen one. In one of their many visits, Mr. Esan said, "whatever you need including money, don't hesitate to ask." Thank you for considering us creditworthy. You are a family friend in need.

ITK catering (Mr. & Mrs. Karimat Ayoade) was always there, and anytime food is ready we send people to pick up and "one day I dropped the change I had with me, and she said "this is the only way I can support," my wife recounted. I cannot thank her and the family enough for all my fish stew, egusi soup, etc. thank you!

Mrs. Bola Adeniyi (Mama Adeniyi), we thank God for your life. We are grateful to you for the many provisions of Akara (bean cake), and pray that God will meet you at your point of need.

Mr. & Mrs. Seun & Bukola Ogunsola, thank you for everything. You went out of your way every time to make my wife and I comfortable all the time. I was discharged from the hospital few days before Thanksgiving and without asking, you dropped a well prepared roasted whole Turkey at my doorstep when we were not home, among very many other supports. Only a very few can be compared to you in your generosity. Thank you so much.

Mr. & Mrs. Kayode & Irene Lano, thank you for your tireless and continuous giving, supports and prayers. May God reward your generosity.

Dr. Onwudiwe – with your visit at the hospital, your many calls, your encouragement and words of advice, you are like a father to us. We appreciate you.

Rev. & Dr. (Mrs.) Kenny & Chidinma – words cannot convey our appreciation for your generousity, supports and prayers. Thank you, may God reward you abundantly.

Dr. & Mrs. Tunji & Victoria Fapojuwo, thank you for your many visits to the hospital and my house, and for checking on us and your continuous prayers.

Pastor & Mrs. Tunde & Bose Aina, thank you for your prayers and words of encouragement, may God continue to bless you and your family.

Mrs. Bunmi Olayinka, thank you for visit, prayers and the worship songs you uploaded for us, they are inspiring, we pray that you will continue to worship the Lamb of Glory.

Mr. & Mrs. Gilles & Clarisse Ngaha – on hearing the news, Giles, you almost jump from UAE to Canada and asked your wife to come immediately. Clarisse, thank you so much. You were the only one who asked if you can come and stay with me at home; I really appreciate it, thank you, may God meet you at the point of your needs.

Mr. & Dr (Mrs.) Wale & Juliet Onabadejo, thank you for your help. Your presence made a lot of difference during my admission in Unit 32 of the Foothills Medical Clinic. Uncle Wale, thank you for the different types of natural fruits and vegetable drinks you showed us.

Mr. & Mrs. Joseph & Grace Oyelusi, thank you for your many visits to the hospital and to our house, and for your words of encouragement.

Pastors Michael & Bola Oladosu, sharing your life experience and survival story was a big source of encouragement for me. Thank you so much. Your healing shall be permanent in Jesus Name.

Dr. Sam & Mrs. Tinu Anifowose, you are one of our first family friends since we arrived in Canada about two decades ago. You are also the first to introduce us to SourSop line of products to complement the medical treatments. You are a true friend. Thank you so much for your support and prayers.

Mr. & Mrs. Isaac & Adenike Olagundoye, thank you for your visits to the hospital and to our house, and for your words of encouragement. Even with daddy's health, he was still able to visit us, thank you so much!

Mr. & Mrs. Tumi Aderibigbe, thank you so much for encouraging me to journal my experience, without which this book would not have been this detailed. We thank God for your lives for praying and encouraging us through prayers and worship songs.

Ms. Kikelomo Adekoya and Mrs. Obilana – thank you for sharing your experiences as caregiver and patient, we were encouraged when we attended your thanksgiving and pray that your healing will be permanent.

Mr. Sam & Mrs. Marie Akinsanya, Mr. Ben Ezenta, Mr. & Mrs. Gbalajobi, Mr. & Mrs. Taiwo Johnson, Mr. & Mrs. Austin Omobhude, Mr. Moses Ojemakinde, Dr. & Mrs. Carlton & Ijenna Osakwe, Dr. & Mrs. Chika Onwekuwe, Mrs. Dorothy Thompson, Dr. Joseph Osuji, Pastor & Mrs. Eddy Udofia, Mrs. Remi Dumade, Mr. &

Mrs. Bayo Okunlola, Chief & Mrs. Bisi Adedeji, Mr. & Mrs. Edward Ogum, Mrs. Biola Sobowale, Pastor & Mrs. Bosun Akinde, Mr. & Mrs. Samuel Adeyinka, Dr. Bayo Olowe, Mr. Fred Prince, Mr. Kayode Idris, Mr. & Mrs. Femi & Becky Farinu, Mr. & Mrs. Kunle & Kemi Adeyemi, Mrs. Wumi Ogunlele (South), Mrs. Bisi Jagunna, Mr. & Mrs. Toyin & Bukky Okelana, Mrs. Biola Omipidan, Mrs. Flora Utunedi, Mrs. Yemi Okikiolu, Mr. & Mrs. Adebusola Oni (RCCG Christ Embassy), Pastor Toks Balogun RCCG Rehoboth Assembly, Pastor & Mrs. Segun Shitta-Bey, Mrs. Osazele, Pastors Lemmy & Oyinda Unuigbe, members of RCCG House of David, Calgary and other parishes of RCCG, and many others who came to visit at home and at the hospital and those who called, thank you for your support, your words of encouragement and most importantly, for your prayers.

Pastor & Mrs. Tanyi & Sally Adelbert, Apostle Elhadj Diallo, Mr. & Mrs. Chris & Sarah Nwachukwu, Mr. Ben Ezeigbo thank you for your supports, visits, advice, words of encouragement and prayers.

Mr. (Pastor) Thompson Ehimowo, though you did not know I was sick or had cancer, you went out of your way to search for us because you needed to deliver a message from God. Indeed, you were a harbinger of good news because the message from God to me was that "my body is a sanctuary of God, and therefore, I shall not die but live." That message was not only an encouragement, but also a confirmation of similar messages from other people. Thank you for your visits and prayers.

The Mosuro family, Olamide, Kunle & Oyinda Ibrahim, Tomiwa and Mr. & Mrs. Mosuro, thank you for your visits, words of encouragements, supports and your prayers. Thank you Olamide for making time out of your busy schedule to see how I am doing whenever you visit Calgary, thank you, may God continue to prosper your way.

Pastor & Mrs. Sunny Adeniyi, thank you for your prayers and your many calls. May God continue to strengthen you.

Pastor & Mrs. Kayode & Mrs. Lanle Ajayi, thank you for your concerns, efforts and prayers, even when your general overseer (Rev. (Dr.) Mike Okonkwo) visited Calgary in 2016.

Pastor & Pastor (Mrs.) Samuel & Olufunke Ilesanmi (RCCG Christ Love Assembly): Thank you for your prayers and words of encouragements. You always say "we are in it together." Whenever you had special program, you brought your guests ministers to pray with us – including Pastor Adeniji the RCCG North America Prayer Coordinator. It was a surprise visit, and I thank you for making time to pray for me out of your tight schedules; and Pastor Femi Olawale, RCCG Canada Coordinator - thank you for coming to our house to offer prayers, we appreciate you.

Rev, Moses Adekola, Dr. & Mrs. Afolayan, Mr. Femi & Mrs.. Idiono Adepoju, Mr. & Mrs. Victor Fagbola, Mr. & Mrs. Funmi Omidele, Mrs. Lara Aderibigbe, Mr. Conrad Aglah, Mr.& Mrs. Jide & Busola Ayotade, Mr. Larry Udeani, Mrs. Florence Odiakosa, Mr. Zik Obianwa, Mr. Ifedi Obianwa, Mr. Goodluck Nwaerondu, Pastors Sunday & Kemi Micho, Ms. Faith Greaves, Mrs. Debra Sanni, Aunty Theresa (TK), Dr. & Mrs. Chiwetelu, Ms. Ada Duru, Mr. Innocent Ighalo, Mr. & Mrs. Sola Oduga, Mr. & Mrs. Olawale, Mr. & Mrs. Opeodu, Ms. Ruth Adekunle, Mr. Adeolu Shobowale, Mr. Peter Atole,. Thank you for your calls, visits, supports and prayers. We appreciate you very much

Mr. & Mrs. Bunmi and Bola Adetula thank you for your care and prayers. Through you we came in contact with Pastor Sunday Abidogun of the Gospel Faith Mission in Calgary and Pastor & Pastor (Mrs.) Akinola from Nigeria who came to our home during their visit to Calgary. Thank you all for your prayers and supports.

Rev. & Pastor (Mrs.) Bible Davis, thank you for all your prayers, even though you were not around, you took the time to call on a conference bridge; thank you.

Mr. Osita Nwofor, Mr. Ben Okafor, Mr. Steve Anene, thank you for your concerns, even though you heard very late.

Mr. Mike Redeker Vice President and CIO Canadian Pacific Railway, Mr. & Mrs. Mbanugo, Mr. & Mrs. Tony & Seyi Arthur, Ms Shannon Pate, Pastor & Mrs. Eddy Udofia, Mr. Don Morgan, members of the Toastmaster 9901 (Station 29) club and my colleagues and friends at Canadian Pacific Railway, thank you for supports and for being part of my recovery and my second chance.

Ochuko and Mercy (Ofiuvwo), and Joseph and John (Ogunleye) are some of my "children" who insisted that their parents brought them to see me in the hospital bed. With them around, life takes a different meaning all the time. I thank God for your lives, for your parents, and for having you around. God will uphold you and bring his purposes to your lives to fruition.

The staff of The UPS Store #45 – Rifat Khandokah, Navdeep Kaur, Cylena Cruikshank, Allen Dispo, thank you for running and managing the office, we cannot thank you enough.

Mr. & Mrs. Andrew & Kemi Frid, thank you for always being there for us, you are one of those we can call upon anytime, may God continue to bless you abundantly.

Rev. Chudi Nato: Thank you for your visit, encouragement and prayers. May your anointing never run down.

A special mention is required for the following mostly out of town family members, pastors and friends for their concerns, prayers, advice and support:

My big brother, Pastor Debo Oladele, who left his family to be with us for six good months and his wife in Nigeria, Mrs. Doja Oladele; my immediate big brother and his wife Mr. Adenle & Mrs. Tayo Oladele, my dear brother and doctor Dr. Rotimi & Mrs. Funmi Oladele, and my only sister and her husband, Pastor Rufus & Mrs. Sade Akinwale, and Pastor Toye Oladele. Thank you for your prayers and faith in God.

My in-laws, Pastor & Pastor (Mrs.) Isaac & Florence Adekule, Mr. Kayode Shobowale, Mr. & Mrs. Tunde & Banke Shobowale, Mr. Wasiu Fatoyinbo, Mr. Femi Sobowale, Mrs. Seyi Idowu, Deborah and our dear sister and friend, Mrs.

149

Remi Oyefeso, thank you for your concerns and your prayers.

Pastor Abiodun Coker and your friend from Saskatoon – Pastor Kola and Pastor & Mrs. Ayeni from RCCG Brooks, Alberta, Canada, thank you for your prayers and for making the time to visit my wife and I all the way from the USA. We appreciate you, your wife and your entire family.

Pastor Abiodun Doherty (Australia), despite the significant difference in time, you always make sure to call us at our convenient time. We appreciate you and your family for your concerns, continuous follow-up and prayers.

Mr. Ben Moloud Edmonton, thank you for your concerns, prayers, supports and always checking on us.

Through Pastor Abi-Abiola, I met Pastor Olawoyin who was in Calgary, visiting his children. Pastor Olawoyin took me like a son and committed his time to praying for me and my wife. We appreciate you for what God is doing in your life. I also met two other out of town men of God through Pastor Abi-Abiola. Thank you again, Pastor Abi-Abiola for all your efforts and care. Whenever you had guest pastors, you always bring them to our house or the hospital – including Pastor Fela Keshinro from Winnipeg and Prophet Moses Iyanda from Nigeria, we cannot thank you enough. We pray that the anointing of God in your life will not run dry.

Mrs. Abiola (UK), though a fighter and survivor, you did not let your situation bogged you down. You saw your experience and condition as a means to an end and not an end in itself and used the opportunities to minister words of wisdom whenever we have time to talk. May God perfect His work in your life.

Pastor Kayode Olufunmilayo at the Redemption Camp in Lagos Nigeria, thank you for your prayers and concerns, we pray God will perfect all that concerns you and your family.

Pastor Sam Elijah (USA), Evangelist Belema Alibi – Holy Ghost Fellowship, USA, Mrs. Remi Yahaya (FCET, Akoka, Lagos), thank you for all your supports and prayers.

I also like to espress my gratitude to Michael D Robin, Kay Hannan, Nichole Resciniti, Jg Walz, members of the Radiatory and Esoteric Healing group of Morya Federation and others for your thoughts and prayers. Thank you.

My gratitude goes to the following group of people for their professionalism, dedication and encouragements.

- The Emergency doctors, nurses and staff of FMC
- Dr. S.A. Workun, the nurses, staff and members of Unit 32 of FMC
- The various doctors, nurses, technicians and staff of the Special Services and different laboratories
- My oncologist and hematologist Dr. Peter Duggan and his able secretary and nurse Ms Arika Rohrick. Dr. Nancy Zacarias, Ms. Judith Olesen – Transplant Coordinator, and others thank you!
- The doctors, pharmacists, nurses and staff of the Multiple Myeloma clinic, Chemotherapy Medical Day Care Unit, the Blood and Marrow Transplant (BMT) Clinic, the Apheresis Clinic, and the unit 57 team
- Psychosocial, the OASIS and other groups and clinics of Tom Baker Cancer Centre (TBCC)
- The doctors, pharmacists, nurses and staff of Home Parental Therapy Program (HPTP)
- Dr. S.A. Walji, my family doctor and the nurses.

I also like to thank my employer Canadian Pacific Railway, for providing a good working environment and benefits that allowed me to go through this ordeal with minimal financial stress, and to my boss and colleagues for your understanding.

TO GOD BE THE GLORY!

From our Reviewers

We have the privilege of reading an excerpt from the book titled, "Second Chance   Surviving the Battles of Cancer" from a family who passed through the valley of the shadow of death but with faith in the Lord Jesus (OUR HEALER) and with the care received from the doctors was able to defeat death. Thisbook will give inspiration and hope to other people battling with life threatening diseases. What an inspiration to keep fighting the good fight of faith. We recommend this book for everyone. To God be the glory. The name of the Lord is truly a strong tower. Be encouraged as you read this great testimony.

Pastors Ademola & Iheoma Farinu
(RCCG - VICTORY CHAPEL, VICTORIA BC, CANADA

*   *   *

As I read through this section, I could not help but reflect on how Bayo put his trust in God through this very difficult journey in his life. As I visited him in the hospital or in his home, there was always someone praying for him and his wife, Yinka. At times, when it looked so bleak, there was hope that only God could bring him through the pain, even when the outcome was not always clear. I am reminded of the verse in scripture from Hebrews 11: 1 " Now faith is confidence in what we hope for and assurance about what we do not see." As you read through the pages of this book, you will read of a man and his family who lived this verse, and who trusted God completely with his life.

Rev. Noral Woodburn,
Pastor, BP Church, Calgary Canada

* * *

The second chance is a book written by a friend, and teaches about the significance of taking advantage of making a decision when confronted with life unexpected surprise. The writer actually, suddenly, fell ill and by the grace of God, took the right action and with the faith in God, he is now telling the tales of his life.

People should never be condemned to death due to any type of ailment, most especially, cancer disease, due to the fact that medicine has progressed beyond what the masses knew about. It was exactly the same story before the discovery of penicillin, and I strongly believe that the power of prayer has guided the doctors to diagnose the best solution for the writer. This explained why God is the most and essential part of our beings. Things happen, but those who live under the shelter of the Almighty will always be protected.

I have personally known the writer for almost 17 years, and has always been in good health until suddenly, the news of his sickness broke out and according to the book; series of action and reaction occurs which has led to immediate treatment, rather than waiting for further consultations. I regard this as the handmaiden of the omnipotence.

Today, the writer is doing well, and is going about his daily life. We are joyful with him and the family. It is written, God will never give you a test that is above you. I will encourage anyone who desires to be motivated in life should lay hands on this book.

Dr. Sam & Mrs. Tinu Anifowose
Family Friend, Calgary, Alberta, Canada

* * *

Bayo Oladele is an IT Guru. He clearly explains and recounts the details of his journey as a cancer survivor.

Presented as a simple, easy-to-read-and-understand story, Bayo's experience is divided into four (4) parts:

The first part talks about people's general perception of cancer, what cancer really is, and what cancer professionals have to say about cancer.

- The second part is the events before his journey, the discovery and his diagnosis
- The third part entails his diagnosis, and the decision to start cancer treatments
- The fourth part entails the beginning of his treatment and beyond

Based on our close proximity to the family and as eyewitnesses to some of the events, we can attest to the factuality of this book. We give glory to God for His infinite mercies and sparing Bayo's life to be able to share his story.

This book is an empowering life story, and a must read for enlightenment about what cancer really is, and how it is perceived by those who have or had it.

Daniel & Marian Ofiuvwo,
Family Friend, Calgary, Alberta

* * *

Nobody knows when something as deadly as cancer will attack. As a survivor, dedicated to supporting people during their treatments and recovery journey, first and foremost, I am thankful to God for Bayo and Yinka, for setting a precedent in the community by breaking off the stigma on cancer attack. It was quite impressive how they called for support and avoided secrecy. This book is a proof. Journeying with the Oladeles was another opportunity to experience God and His Almighty-ness, and, to experience their 'Faith at work,' as they allowed their Faith to cast a divine shadow over the reality of the cancer attack.

As they collaborated with the health care practitioners, they engaged in prayer sessions, declarations and decrees from the Bible, praise and worship sessions, question/answer sessions, visitations, special prayer/counseling ministry, and many practical ways that enhanced recovery. Giving up was not an option. Giving in to the 'suffering' was not a choice. The only option was survival and victory! The prayer is that 'affliction will not return' to Bayo, his household and all. The hope is that readers will be encouraged, strengthened and delivered from this deathly attack called Cancer.

God is good!
Dr. Adeyinka & Oluyinka Marcus

* * *

Myeloma. That's the one word in my iPhone note for 2016-04-02. I assumed Yinka was calling to wish me a happy birthday. Instead, she said, "I need you here," and hung up.

Cancer. Chemo. X-ray. Those words were coming up again! I had heard it repeatedly in the last two years. It was a painful news but it no longer felt like a death sentence. Two other friends were winning the battle.

Thank you so much for sharing your experience, and especially emphasizing the fact that cancer is not a death sentence. I often describe you as an open book, and sharing your journey with cancer in this book attest to it.

God bless.
Mr. & Mrs. Tumi & Kike Aderibigbe

* * *

This book is very far, reaching with facts about cancer, particularly coming from a survivor. When Bayo and Sis Yinka told us about the disease, they were also quick to mention that was the fact and not the truth. When we sensed the force of the faith that was coming from both of them, my wife and I could do nothing less than join our faith with theirs to release the power of God over the situation, and thank God we did.

We are not surprised of Bro Bayo's victory over cancer; we are just amazed at the awesomeness of God. We had an assurance that the Word of God would never fail, and it did not. According to 1 John 5:4, the victory that overcomes the world is our faith. We will like to congratulate the family for the defeat of cancer in the life of our Brother, glory be to God!

Pastors Fola and Sunny Adeniyi
Senior Pastors/Co-founders
Joy Overflow International Church, Calgary.

* * *

Everybody agrees life is precious. So much is done by the society to ensure that life could be enjoyed to the full. Medical facilities, new research findings continue to seek answers to threats posed by so many diseases that may cut short life and the enjoyment of it.

Cancer is one of those deadliest diseases that claim lives without mercy, and with short notice or no warnings at all. It has become a threat to life that Cancer foundations have been formed in different parts of the world, to step up treatment and save lives. Having cancer is like being face-to-face with a lion. It's victims are like the biblical Daniel who was only saved by divine intervention.

In this book, Mr. Oladele tries to assure readers that being diagnosed for cancer is no confirmation of "death warrant." Hope has risen more these days because of research findings, suggestion to lifestyle changes, medical check-ups to detect cancer early and tackle it.

Mr. Oladele emphasized the need for medical check-ups with the example of the 'providential' suggestion of another X-Ray by an angel of God in the raiment of a medical Doctor! That last X-ray made the difference, which gave him a chance to live!

He attributed his survival to divine intervention, and to medical science. He is especially grateful to God for giving him a second chance to live. Who will not be? Surviving an attack of cancer is like surviving a life-threatening duel with a lion. Warmest congratulations to Mr. Oladele and welcome to our world again!

Mr. & Mrs. Phillip & Olubunmi Latilo
Calgary, Alberta

* * *

"Second Chance – Surviving the Battles of Cancer." is an educative, inspiring and poignant account of the reality of the cell compositions in the human body which are not to be feared, but rather, to be understood.

I appreciate your courage in the fight for your life and the humility to enlighten all of us along the way. I wish you a complete recovery, and a cancer free future....

Mr. & Mrs. Derin & Moji Taiwo
Calgary, Alberta, Canada.

* * *

This book is a must read. Reading from someone with the experience of surviving cancer is paramount in the healing process. As the author indicated, "Oncologist or Cancer" may mean different things to people. Reading about the concepts from a lived experience brings the meaning closer to home while helping to create hope.

According to the author, hearing out about the diagnoses for the first time brought deep thoughts regarding the future. These deep thoughts can be softened with knowledge from someone with the experience. The hope and a sense of positivity seen in the author will be helpful to others because they are vital to healing.

Also important to note in the author's narration is his determination to survive, a sense of perseverance and ability to seek out help. The decision to undertake early treatment made a great difference for him. This book is an enlightening read for anyone hoping to heal.

Mr. & Dr. (Mrs.) Wale & Juliet Onabadejo, RN.

*   *   *

"The Auithor has provided insight to the fact that Faith and Science do not conflict in any way. They are complimentary. Faith takes over where Science stops and God has given us knowledge to use science for the benefits of mankind. This is a must read book".

Mr. & Mrs. Tope & Bola Esan,
Flavours Restaurant,
Calgary, Canada

*   *   *

This book will give you good understanding about cancer disease, steps to its cure and the miraculous testimony of God that is able to heal cancer. As you read it, may the inspiration of the almighty God come upon your spirit to receive life over death –

Pastors Tunde & Bose Aina
The Encounter International
Calgary Canada

*   *   *

Over a decade ago, our path crossed with this family. Their strength beside faith in God is in the quiet demeanor of Mr Oladele and the ever radiant smile of Mrs Oladele. The news of the diagnosis no doubt altered the quiet demeanor and radiant smile but not their trust in the ONE that has the final say about life. Every life experience presents an opportunity to testify. The book is a testimony that reveals the finger of God in the affairs of men. It affirms once again that nothing is not over until it is over. The book shows the relevant place of both social and faith communities in addition to a good healthcare system as we journey through life. We celebrate the victory of this family and gladly recommend the book for your reading or gifting it to a friend in need of encouragement.

Dr. Abiodun & Caroline Coker
Dallas, Texas, USA

* * *

Interesting and educational. The book examples cancer from a family's point of view and the trials and tribulations that go with such a diagnosis. It encourages those who may be diagnosed in the future to fight and believe in God. The information in the book must be shared not only with the Nigerian community in Calgary in particular but the general global population that we can beat cancer. Congratulations to the Oladele's on this venture.

Mr. & Mrs. Wale & Bernie Gbalajobi
Calgary, Canada

* * *

It is a privilege and an honor to give a review of this book.

Second Chances is a remarkable tail of a family's triumphant journey overcoming and rising above the disease that has and continues to claim many lives around us.

We have supported from a distance many people through the battle of cancer, but never did we realize the battle they actually fought behind closed doors.

Reading this book gave us new eye sight similar to one who was blind and now could see.

As we read the words between the lines, a new level of empathy and understanding emerged for those we know that have battled the disease and survived.

How much support they need not just in prayers but in material, physical and emotional too. It also caused an ache in us for those who have passed away knowing how much of a battle they fought.

Thank you Yinka and Bayo for opening our eyes to the untold story of this disease and it's affect on everyone.

Pastors Ben & Dee Adekugbe
Calgary World Harvest Christian Centre &
All Woman Ministry

* * *

After reading the excerpt from "A Second Chance - Surviving the Battles of Cancer", it is obvious that Bayo wrote this book in an effort to aid other cancer patients. This memoir is soul-searching that will in no doubt speak to many who prefer sense to sensibility as resonated in Bayo's matter-of-fact tone. "Second Chance - Surviving the Battles of Cancer" is characteristic of the man himself and it is impossible not to be inspired by Bayo's story and his willingness to share it. Thank you Bayo for doing this.

Mr. & Mrs. Peter & Julie Oganwu,
Calgary, Canada

* * *

In life, everyone will taste moments of wellness and ill-health at one time or the other, regardless of one's spiritual or material status. The rich and the poor, the elites and the down-trodden, the believers and unbelievers, whether living in the developed or under-developed world, it is inevitable.

The most dreaded sickness of this time, this our generation, is cancer and the mere mentioning it instills fear in people. While we administer various medications to cure our ailments, either in medical, orthodox or traditional way, fate goes a long way in whatever is the outcome of our efforts.

I commend the courage of Mr. Bayo and Mrs. Yinka Oladele for sharing their experience with the dreadful cancer. This will go a long way in motivating others to remain hopeful and be strong in the face of any traumatic experience.

I pray that God will make it a permanent cure for you and may He also cure all those who are undergoing any form of ailments at this time.

Thank you.
Alhaji & Alhaja Azeez & Adenike Ola-Ojetola
Calgary, Alberta, Canada

* * *

Permit me to call this book a story of courage and the testimony of how being tough can last tough time. Courage is not absence of fear, but rather the judgment that something else; your faith in God is more important. Courage is a great asset to win life battles be it in the spiritual or the physical. Your exemplary courage even in the face of death helps to conquer the fearsome threat of cancer that it could not touch your mind, heart, and soul though almost take away your physical ability. The disease of cancer has help in discovering the fighter within you. In surviving this gruesome story of cancer, I see the beginning of a beautiful life story start up in you. Note that you are not being given second chance but the beginning of life altogether. I see God telling you that in a while, you have had your fair share of suffering, and that now it's your time to lap up all the happiness that life can offer.

Congratulations, you have found your real family in people who stood by your bedside all this time when you are struggling with chemo.

"The ultimate measure of a man is not where he stands in moments of comfort and convenience, but where he stands at a time of challenge and controversy." – Dr. Martin Luther King Jr.

Samuel & Olufunke Ilesanmi
Pastor, RCCG Christ Love Assembly
Calgary, Alberta, Canada

*   *   *

A comprehensive, dynamic, and eminently practical presentation of the work of grace and the healing powers of Christ.

In this timely unique exploration of Life's unexpected challenges, SECOND CHANCE unveils a simple yet radical truth. With passion and clarity, Bayo and Yinka clearly poured out their hearts so that readers can tackle challenges and obstacles with wisdom, spiritual power and God's authority. They outline these facts;

- Understand your authority in the ministry of healing
- walk out the ministry of healing with anyone you meet and in your personal life
- receive and relay words of knowledge
- implement and apply the word of God to every facet of life

Reading A SECOND CHANCE lays out the biblical rationale for believing that God still wants to heal today, that He still actually heals today, and that He uses people of faith to bring His healing today. The greatest priority, of course, is to nurture one's personal relationship with God and be truly filled with His Spirit.

Pastors Olatubosun & Monisola Sowunmi
RCCG House of David
Calgary, Alberta, Canada

*   *   *

I have known Bayo Oladele and his wife, Yinka for over a decade. Throughout this time, they have always been well, healthy and actively engaged at forefront level in community activities both Nigerian and in Calgary at large. Spiritually, they are active participants in different Christian fellowships, bible study groups and as ushers for many years at our home church, Beddington Pentecostal Church (BP Church).

Given the above, therefore, I was very perplexed when I was invited to their home sometime in April last year, to find a frail-looking Bayo, agonising with a lot of pain on the couch. I was informed about his ongoing battle with the cancer of the bone and plasma cell (bone marrow), a rare cancer disease.

But because of their own selfless support to others in the past and present, Bayo and Yinka received enormous attention and support from the community, both ethnic and the church family. Throughout his several months of treatment, both medical and surgery, they remained strong in their faith amidst fluctuating hope and despair situations. They were firmly anchored and sustained in their faith in the master healer – Jesus., The I Am That I

Am. Hallelluia! Bayo was rescued from the 'jaws' of the master killer and destroyer – cancer!

Given the personalities of Bayo and Yinka in sharing knowledge, materials and spirituality with others and given the community support in their time of trial, it is not surprising they have written this book, not only in the spirit of sharing their experience but above all, to glorify God, the giver and taker of life, for returning Bayo's life, under a circumstance, where the faithless would have lost hope. Glory be to God for ever and ever. Our redeemer liveth! Praise Him forever and ever. Hallelluia

I encourage you all to read and enjoy and support the efforts of Bayo and Yinka, in this masterpiece – written from the hearts. And God bless you as you do so. It was not easy.

Dr. Julius Adekunle & Mrs. Elma Ogunnariwo
Sherwood Gardens
Calgary, Alberta, Canada

*   *   *

"This book has thoroughly documented how to face situation that no one could prepare for. It is remarkable how life could change overnight, how dreams could be turned upside down or delayed and how faith could be tested to it's foundation by a single report. This book is a great resource for the fight of faith, test of friendship and the bond of love. This book would encourage many who are currently on the similar journey to the one documented"

Mr. & Mrs. Seun & Bukola Ogunsola
Calgary, Alberta, Canada

* * *

This book is a bold attempt by Bayo to demystify the scourge called Cancer. It is an invaluable account of a directly affected individual that we should all pay a detailed attention to. I enjoin all to religiously follow all the advice and recommendations therein.

We pray that Almighty Allah protects all of us from all "incurable" diseases currently ravaging the world. May He Almighty endow the human race quickly with sufficient knowledge that will provide permanent cure to all such diseases.

We salute Mr. & Mrs. Oladele's courage to publish this book for the benefit of mankind.

Alhaji & Alhaja Muideen & Basirat Adeyemi
President, Multiplex International Inc.
Calgary, Alberta, Canada

* * *

"The courage, candour and openness with which the Oladeles are dealing with the life-changing event that was thrust upon them without notice, is, in the very least, highly commendable and admirable. I wish them and the care-management team continuing success in dealing with the circumstances, to a very positive conclusion." -

Chief & Chief (Mrs.) Adeniyi & Lolade Akanni
Calgary, Alberta, Canada

*   *   *

Upon reading A Second Chance, one readily concludes that while we need and use the healthcare system, God is the ultimate healer.

We had the privilege of visiting and praying with Bayo and his wife throughout the period of their trial. They never wavered in their faith in God's ability to heal. Bayo and Yinka's journey recounted in this book is a true testament of God's faithfulness in the face of adversity and that God is still very much in the business of healing even in this modern day.

We recommend this book to any one who wants to grow in faith, particularly those who are believing God for healing.

Rev. & Dr. (Mrs.) Kenny Thompson
Voice of Faith and Triumph Ministry
Calgary, Alberta, Canada

* * *

The journey was long but short to the glory of God. It was full of pain physically, emotionally, mentally and spiritually. All through it Bayo stayed strong and his wife (Yinka) was always smiling. This smile was one of the factors that helped Bayo in the healing journey. I learnt soo much from both of them during this journey that "in life what you can't change, accept it with joy and leave the rest to God"

I witnessed Bayo Oladele learning to walk like a baby during the illness but now can take giant steps. There was a period that he could not eat the hospital meals and Yinka would prepared amala from home that would be in form of liquid. Yinka and I would be persuading and encouraging him in a play-way method to eat the meal just as you will encourage a baby learning to eat solid meals. Yinka was a strong woman, dedicated, and stood firmly beside Bayo through the journey. I joked with her that "the hospital would have to give her honourary degree in nursing". Bayo is indeed " a fighter" he fought and conquered the battle called cancer to the glory of God. Glory be to God for been with him and his family. We are eternal grateful O Lord.

Mr. Sina & Mrs. Sola Akinsanya
Calgary, Alberta, Canada

* * *

Blessed be the God and Father of our Lord Jesus Christ, the Father of mercies and God of all comfort, who comforts us in all our tribulations that we may be able to comfort those who are in any trouble with the comfort with which we ourselves are comforted by God. 2 Corinthians 1 vs. 3 - 4.

Therefore, we hope that as you read this book of personal experience and testimony to the goodness of God, you would be encouraged and resolute in your abiding faith in the Lord no matter the vicissitudes of life you might be facing and we pray that your testimony will abide in Jesus Name.

Deacon Michael & Dr. (Mrs.) Lydia Oladosu
Calgary, Alberta, Canada

* * *

My dear Bayo and Yinka,

I must congratulate you for sharing your life experience and journey with everybody in this book. It is indeed very remarkable, encouraging and educational. We also thank God for using you as His ambassador to manifest His work. I am convinced that this book will surely encourage any one passing through same experience. There is always that light at the end of the tunnel provided there is Faith, Strength and Patience to fight that devil.

By publishing this book, you have once again demonstrated your exceptional character of humility and service to mankind. Just as you are always eager to serve and help people, your experience is a manifestation of God's Love for people that truly serve him. He will continue to shower His love, Blessings and Mercies upon you and your family for ever.

Once again, thanks for sharing!

Dr. Theo & Mrs. Uche Okeke
Calgary, Alberta, Canada

*   *   *

Some Questions Answered

Following are some common questions that we have been asked many times by different people. The answers provided are our sincere attempts at addressing these questions based on our experience and information gathered from many places. The answers are our opinions only and do not constitute legal or medical advice. Please consult your doctors and other professional bodies for official answers.

- *What did the doctors say were the cause of your cancer?*

While it is possible to suggest a cause for certain types of cancer, there is no identifiable cause for multiple myeloma.

- *Was your way of life or mode of living responsible for your cancer?*

Again, it is possible that certain cancers may be caused by exposure to certain conditions, there is no specific condition that has been identified to be responsible for MM

- *What could you have done better?*

Considering the above answers, it is therefore difficult to identify what might have been done wrong or what may have prevented it from hapenning.

- *Did yearly medical check-up helped?*

Absolutely! Medical check-up is very good, important and advised. The first indication of MM in my body was discovered through the checkup. Though I got a clean bill of health from the provincial cancer board, the provincial cancer test was focused on prostate cancer for men over 50 years.

- *What advice do you have for others about healthy living?*

Healthy living should not be a matter of debate. Regardless of whether or not cancer may be caused by the way we live, both common sense and studies have shown that healthy living makes healthy person. It is abosolutely important that we live healthy life.

- *What is your view about the modern medicine on Cancer treatment?*

The difference between modern medicine and traditional is that the modern way is scientifically proving with practical evidence and systematic way of dispensing dosages.

- *Are you open to people contacting you?*
  - *To talk about their challenges*
  - *For spiritual advice*
  - *For one on one consultation?*
  - *To pray together?*

People have asked us these and many other similar questions.

We will be happy and humbled to meet with anyone or group for:

- Speaking engagements
- Visit to churches, congregations, communities and groups
- Seminars
- Workshops

We will also be on book signing tour. Please check our website for details.

www.oladele.ca
secondchance@oladele.ca
mysecondchancetolive@gmail.com

Healing Together
Through Sharing

We have been treamendously blessed by God and people that God placed around us. Our families, friends, colleagues, groups, communities and churches and people of God all over have prayed and supported us materially, emotionally and spiritually. We have never been left out without help.

We have decided to give back as much as we can and as much as possible. Much has been given to us and much is expected from us.

If you are a survivor or a fighter and need someone to talk to; If you are a caregiver and you are feeling alone or lonely and over burdened; If you are a family member or friend of a fighter or survivor and you need someone to discuse with, we are happy to inform you that the authors can be reached at the following contacts for:

- Advice and encouragements
- Discussions
- Consultations
- Prayers

To obtain a copy

You can obtain your hard copy or copies of

SECOND CHANCE
Surviving the battles of cancer

at

amazon

www.oladele.ca

The book is also available online and worldwide in

Ebook & Kindle Formats

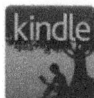

Review and Feedback

WE WOULD APPRECIATE YOUR REVIEW, FEEDBACK OR COMMENTS REGARDING THIS BOOK:

Please send your comments to:

secondchance@oladele.ca
mysecondchancetolive@gmail.com

You can also review online at

www.amazon.ca or www.oladele.ca

Please note that some of the reviews will be placed on our social media, if you do not want your name online, please advice.

REFERENCES

[1] http://www.who.int/cancer/en/
[2] http://www.worldcancerday.org/about
[3] https://en.wikipedia.org/wiki/Cancer
[4] http://cancer-code-europe.iarc.fr/index.php/en/about-cancer/whatis-cancer
[5] https://www.aacrfoundation.org/Pages/what-is-cancer.aspx
[6] https://en.wikipedia.org/wiki/Cell_growth
[7] http://www.cancer.ca/en/cancer-information/cancer-101/what-is-cancer/cancer-cell-development/?region=on
[8] http://wellcommons.com/weblogs/health-beat/2011/apr/1/we-all-carry-cancer-cells-last-part-we-c/
[9] http://www.menshealth.com/health/it-true-we-all-have-cancer-cells
[10] https://en.wikipedia.org/wiki/Multiple_myeloma#cite_note-WCR2014Cp513-3
[11] https://www.cancer.org/cancer/multiple-myeloma/causes-risks-prevention/what-causes.html
[12] http://www.cancer.ca/en/cancer-information/cancer-type/multiple-myeloma/multiple-myeloma/?region=on
[13] https://en.wikipedia.org/wiki/Cancer#Causes
[14] http://www.wikilectures.eu/index.php/Cancer_Cells_Char-acteristics
[15] http://www.biology-pages.info/C/Cancer.html
[16] https://www.quora.com/Do-cancer-cells-already-exist-in-the-human-body
[17] http://www.who.int/ionizing_radiation/research/iarc/en/
[18] https://ntp.niehs.nih.gov/results/areas/index.html
[19] https://en.oxforddictionaries.com/definition/growth
[20] https://www.cancer.org/cancer/all-cancer-types.html
[21] https://www.cancer.gov/types
[22] https://en.wikipedia.org/wiki/List_of_cancer_types
[23] http://tbccintegrative.com/

24 http://www.cancer.ca/en/cancer-information/cancer-101/what-is-cancer/?region=on
25 https://www.cancer.org/cancer/all-cancer-types.html
26 https://www.cancer.org/cancer/cancer-basics/signs-and-symptoms-of-cancer.html
27 https://www.merriam-webster.com/dictionary/sign
28 http://www.cancerresearchuk.org/about-cancer/cancer-symptoms#accordion_symptoms2
29 https://www.cancer.gov/about-cancer/diagnosis-staging/symptoms
30http://www.who.int/gho/publications/world_health_statistics/2017/en/
31http://www.albertahealthservices.ca/cancer/cancer.aspx
32http://www.albertahealthservices.ca/info/facility.aspx?id=1007362
33 http://www.cpr.ca/en/careers/why-work-at-cp/compensation-and-benefits
34 https://www.caring.com/articles/activities-of-daily-living-what-are-adls-and-iadls
35 https://en.wikipedia.org/wiki/Activities_of_daily_living
36http://www.albertahealthservices.ca/info/facility.aspx?id=1007362&service=1073213
37 https://www.cancer.org/cancer/multiple-myeloma/detection-diagnosis-staging/staging.html
38 http://www.cancer.ca/en/cancer-information/diagnosis-and-treatment/tests-and-procedures/central-venous-catheter/?region=on
39 http://www.cancer.ca/en/cancer-information/diagnosis-and-treatment/tests-and-procedures/peripherally-inserted-central-catheter/?region=on
40 https://www.cancer.gov/types/myeloma/hp/myeloma-treatment-pdq
41 https://www.spine-health.com/treatment/back-surgery/description-kyphoplasty-surgery